ONE WEEK LOAN
UNIVERSITY OF GLAMORGAN
TREFOREST LEARNING RESOURCES CENTRE
Pontypridd, CF37 1DL
Telephone: (01443) 482626
Books are to be returned on or before the last date below

spatial epidemiology

London Papers in Regional Science

ꝐPion Limited, 207 Brondesbury Park, London NW2 5JN

edited by R.W.Thomas · London papers in regional science 21 · a pion publication

spatial epidemiology

⟁ Pion Limited, 207 Brondesbury Park, London NW2 5JN

© 1990 Pion Limited

British Library Cataloguing in Publication Data
A CIP catalogue record for this book is available from the British Library.

ISBN 0 85086 148 9

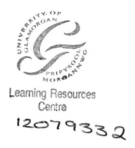

Printed in Great Britain by Page Bros (Norwich) Limited

Contributors

A D Cliff
: *Department of Geography, University of Cambridge, Cambridge CB2 3BU, England*

P Diggle
: *Department of Mathematics, Lancaster University, Lancaster LA1 4YB, England*

A K Dutt
: *Department of Geography and Urban Studies, The University of Akron, Akron, OH 44325, USA*

H M Dutta
: *Department of Biological Sciences, Kent State University, Kent, OH 44242, USA*

A C Gatrell
: *Department of Geography, Lancaster University, Lancaster LA1 4YB, England*

J A Giggs
: *Department of Geography, University of Nottingham, Nottingham NG7 2RD, England*

M Greenberg
: *Department of Urban Studies and Community Health, Rutgers University, New Brunswick, NJ 08903, USA*

P Haggett
: *Department of Geography, University of Bristol, Bristol BS8 1SS, England*

A A Lovett
: *School of Environmental Sciences, University of East Anglia, Norwich NR4 7TJ, England*

D Miller
: *Department of Geography and Urban Studies, The University of Akron, Akron, OH 44325, USA*

S Openshaw
: *Centre for Urban and Regional Development Studies, University of Newcastle upon Tyne, Newcastle upon Tyne NE1 7RU, England*

S Scobie
: *School of Geography, University of Manchester, Manchester M13 9PL, England*

M R Smallman-Raynor
: *Department of Geography, University of Cambridge, Cambridge CB2 3BU, England*

R W Thomas
: *School of Geography, University of Manchester, Manchester M13 9PL, England*

R Wakeford

Health Statistics Group, British Nuclear Fuels plc, Risley, Warrington WA3 6AS, England

D Wartenberg

Robert Wood Johnson Medical School, University of Medicine and Dentistry of New Jersey, Piscataway, NJ 08854–5635, USA

Contents

Introduction: Issues in Spatial Epidemiology

R W THOMAS
University of Manchester

1 Objectives

The words 'spatial' and 'epidemiology' often appear in quite close proximity in medical writing, but examples of their use in conjunction are much rarer (Mayer, 1988). In this volume the term spatial epidemiology is used to describe studies of disease causation and prevention which adopt a distinctly analytical spatial perspective. The sophistication of the analysis may vary from statistical description to formal mathematical analysis, and will often depend on the extent to which the aetiology of the disease in question is understood. Given this brief, the papers contained in this volume have been brought together both to demonstrate the current scope of the subject and to illustrate the range of analytical procedures involved.

Much of the material used was presented to the European Congress of the Regional Science Association held at St John's College, Cambridge, in August 1989. Seven of the papers published here were read to sessions on Spatial Epidemiology at this Congress, the remainder have been commissioned to provide a greater breadth of subject matter.

Mention of regional science begs the natural question about the relationship of spatial epidemiology to a subject which promotes regional analysis within economics, geography, and planning. Hopefully, the connections will become self-evident on reading the individual contributions. However, it is worth emphasising that both subjects share common interests in spatial interaction theory, statistical estimation, equilibrium conditions, and threshold mechanisms. These ideas will surface again later, but here the immediate priority is to set the contributions in context by an examination of the evolving scope and content of spatial epidemiology within its supporting disciplines.

2 Evolution

Links between geography and epidemiology have a long history which Gould (1985) describes as the 'old partnership'. Nevertheless, this relationship has not always proved fruitful, and there have been occasions when geographers have made few contributions to the understanding of disease causation. This patchiness may be attributed to the rather one-sided nature of the 'partnership' whereby, historically, geographers have managed to gain a secure research interest only when a disease at the forefront of epidemiological investigation has had a strong environmental component postulated for its aetiology.

This tendency is illustrated by events during the second half of the
19th century. The mapping of infectious diseases was an established
method of research (Gilbert, 1958), which culminated in Snow's (1855)
map of cholera incidence around the Broad Street pump in Soho,
demonstrating the water-borne transmission of the disease. Such
pioneering examples of spatial epidemiology were brought to a sudden
halt by Pasteur's confirmation of germ theory, and the subsequent
isolation of the parasitic agents responsible for the major infectious
diseases. In the wake of these discoveries, it was thought that little was
to be gained from mapping diseases with known aetiologies.

Contemporary sources (Jones and Moon, 1987; Meade et al, 1988)
attribute the revival of modern medical geography to the French physician
Jacques May (1950; 1960). He reemphasised the environmental influence
by proposing the study of disease ecology, and received acclaim for his
investigation of deficiency diseases in the developing world. His efforts
did much to stimulate a trickle of largely individual research in the 1950s
and 1960s, which had become a torrent by the 1980s. Medical geography
was established on firm foundations, which is now illustrated by its
regular forum in journals like *Social Science and Medicine* and by the
constant appearance of new textbooks (Haynes, 1987; Meade et al, 1988;
Pyle, 1979) and research monographs (Cliff et al, 1986; Greenberg,
1983; Smith and Giggs, 1988).

This expansion of medical geography has undoubtedly opened up new
areas of research. Yet, Meade et al (1988, page 324) have suggested
that an unwanted side effect of this growth has been the division of the
subject into the study of health and disease, and the more recent concern
with health care delivery systems.

A second development has been the emergence of studies which do
not necessarily invoke standard biomedical explanations for disease
causation. Jones and Moon (1987) have argued for a constructionalist
interpretation where the explanation and treatment of disease are regarded
as societal beliefs, not medical facts. They allude to Illich (1975) and
his notion of *iatrogenesis*—the damage to health done by medicine itself.
A related theme has been the interpretation of traditional forms of
medicine as ethnomedical systems; a term which embraces self-treatment,
popular therapies, and the role of faith healers. Good (1986) has drawn
on examples from Africa, where medical pluralism is extensive, to compare
the effectiveness of these systems with those of 'Western' medicine.

Research into alternative forms of medical practice does provide a
fresh geographical perspective. Nevertheless, the emphasis on treatment
and social context, at the expense of causation and prevention, is likely
to place a strain on the 'old partnership' between geography and
epidemiology. This tension arises because alternative medicine sets an
open agenda for medical geography, where no obvious priority is set for
the diseases to be investigated. Epidemiological principles stress

causation and prevention, and so offer the geographer a sharper focus where the investigation is directed at diseases with unknown, or poorly understood, aetiologies. In addition, an understanding of causation provides the building blocks for the construction of forecasting models (Bailey, 1975) and the subsequent evaluation of strategies for disease control—subjects which both have important spatial dimensions.

In the discussion so far we have examined the fortunes of spatial epidemiology within the confines of medical geography. Equally relevant are the evolving principles and practices of epidemiology (Barker, 1982; Barker and Rose, 1984), which have a critical influence on the conduct of research.

A convenient starting point is the idea that each disease must have a singular and specific cause; a notion which followed the discovery of bacterial agents at the end of the last century. This idea was expressed in Koch's postulates which, for some time, provided the guidelines for identifying the agents of infectious disease. Yet, modern experience has shown that the control of infectious disease owes as much to knowledge of contributory factors as it does to vaccination for a specific agent.

Hutt and Burkitt (1986) make the important comment that most contemporary, chronic, noninfectious diseases, including all forms of cancer, are recognised to be the result of a causal chain of events, often occurring over a long period of time. In this scheme, disease in the individual is viewed as a complex interaction between heredity and the environment which operates throughout life. A further complication to the specific-agent explanation arises because most chronic diseases, including those which create high rates of mortality, affect only a small proportion of those who live in the same environment. Thus control programmes designed to protect against harmful environmental and genetic influences will waste resources on many individuals who are not at risk, and may not necessarily increase the life expectancy of these individuals.

The failure to identify specific causes for modern chronic diseases, particularly for cancers, has led to the development of more flexible epidemiological practices. Cancer research has tended to split between experimental research on tumour production, and statistical studies of cancer in human populations (Hutt and Burkitt, 1986). Models of cancer have been dominated by experimental work, which has greatly enhanced knowledge of the final stages of tumour development. However, it is generally recognised that a much greater integration of laboratory and environmental analyses is required if the complete pathways along which cancers develop are to be understood. This switch to less mechanical modes of explanation should also allay some of the fears expressed by the critics of the biomedical model (Dubos, 1959; McKeown, 1979).

3 Context

The contributions to this volume have been collected together to represent contemporary themes in spatial epidemiology. In the first instance, these themes relate to major areas of medical inquiry such as the origins of human cancers, the threat posed by the acquired immunodeficiency syndrome (AIDS), and the treatment and care of mental illness. Moreover, the diversity of questions surrounding these topics has brought about the development of distinctive analytical procedures to tackle their individual characteristics, and provides a secondary technical theme. In this section, I shall examine these topics in their broader contexts to give a background to the individual contributions to this book.

Human cancers are arguably the greatest modern medical challenge yet, although generations of researchers have probed their origins, specific agents have been identified for only a few subtypes. The aetiologies that have been proposed are varied, and implicate environmental carcinogens, viral agents, and genetic factors. The most incisive findings have more often concerned prevention and control, and include the association between tobacco smoking and lung cancer (Doll and Peto, 1976), and the benefits of regular screening for cervical cancer (Hutt and Burkitt, 1986).

One of the first ways in which medical geographers managed to contribute to the debate about the origins of cancer was through mapping their rates of incidence both at national and at international scales (Howe, 1977). Quite often the interpretation of the maps was conflicting. For example, it has been demonstrated that the indigenous population of Japan experience higher rates of stomach cancer than Japanese migrants living in the USA, an observation which implies a dietary component to the aetiology. Nevertheless, the rate of incidence in these migrants is still significantly greater than that experienced by the US white population, indicating the possible role of genetic factors.

The mapping of cancer incidence has prompted some valuable questions and hypotheses about causation. Unfortunately, choropleth mapping can often give a misleading impression of the actual distribution of disease. This ambiguity is a consequence of the 'modifiable areal unit problem' (Openshaw, 1977), which is the recognition that map pattern can vary dramatically if the size and shape of the areal units forming the study region are altered.

It is now much more common to map each case as a point location and to analyse statistical properties of the distribution by using pattern recognition techniques similar to those originally developed in ecology and astronomy (Thomas, 1981). In epidemiological investigation a popular method has been to test case distributions for space-time clustering (Knox, 1963; 1964) which, if significant, is evidence for either a source (or sources) of carcinogens within the study region, or a transmissible disease agent. Such tests, which analyse the distribution of all possible pairs of cases in space and time, cannot distinguish alone between these 2 sources of clustering. However, clinical evidence might point to the more appropriate explanation.

A natural extention to the general screening of cancers for space-time clustering (Mangoud et al, 1985) is to devise more precisely specified statistical models that test directly for case clustering around a suspected source of carcinogens. This approach is dealt with in detail later on. However, it may be noted that some of the most controversial results have concerned the distribution of cases of childhood leukaemia around nuclear power stations and their waste disposal plants (Openshaw et al, 1988). Experience has shown that when such tests are sufficiently targeted at the source, a significant result will raise questions concerning corporate responsibility and environmental safety which extend beyond the statistical implications for causation. The degree to which such statistical results are to be believed has become a key debate in spatial epidemiology, which often revolves around the power of the test in question.

This emphasis on the role of statistical models requires a note of caution, because it is unlikely that a single model is able to accommodate all the facets of the distribution of a cancer. An illustration is provided by the distribution of Burkitt's lymphoma (Burkitt, 1969). The incidence of this cancer is almost exclusively restricted to children in Africa, and its infectious aetiology was suggested by significant space-time clustering amongst cases. Subsequently, the tumors of the lymphoma were shown to be promoted by the Epstein-Barr virus (Epstein and Achong, 1979) in conjunction with the malarial cycle. Yet this confirmed aetiology does not help explain why Burkitt's lymphoma has such a low incidence in countries like India, where both the Epstein-Barr virus and the relevant malarial parasite (*Plasmodium falciparum*) are present in abundance. In other words, the spatial variation is not consistent with the aetiology.

Cancer research has long and established traditions; however, the appearance of AIDS in the 1970s (Dutt et al, 1987) is stimulating new avenues of investigation. Inadvertently, the beginnings of the epidemic coincided with geographical interest in forecasting the spread of infectious diseases (Cliff et al, 1981; 1986; Thomas, 1988) and, given the virulence of the human immunodeficiency virus (HIV), it might have been expected that detailed space-time forecasting would have formed an important element of the control strategy. However, this task has been hampered by the composition of the groups most at risk to HIV infection (homosexual men, intravenous drug misusers, and haemophiliacs); the members of these groups, for reasons of confidentiality, are unlikely to be the most willing subjects of sociospatial enumeration. Aggregative regional statistics are made available in the United Kingdom (CDSC, 1988), but essential information for detailed forecasting, such as the addresses of carriers (HIV positive) and their contacts, is unlikely to be accessible in the short term. If such data problems persist, then current trends point to the development of generalised models for AIDS (Knox, 1986) and the reconstruction of the epidemic from fragmentary sources (Smallman-Raynor and Cliff, 1990). An alternative approach is found in social medicine where survey methods have been used to monitor the effects of preventative measures (such as modifications to sexual behaviour) on the incidence of HIV infection among homosexual men (Carne et al, 1987).

Investigation of the origins of human cancers is helped by the knowledge that their symptoms are usually well defined, which implies their diagnosis will be reliable. In contrast, the diagnosis of mental illness is much more problematic. Most psychiatric disorders are not supported by confirmed aetiologies, and their symptoms are not confined to a single diagnostic category. Given this uncertainty, it is not surprising to learn that misdiagnosis is quite a common event (Weiner and Del Gaudio, 1976); a defect which imbues psychiatric data with a fuzziness that obscures its statistical interpretation.

Despite these difficulties, a variety of aetiologies have been suggested for most psychiatric disorders. There is some fragmentary evidence that genetic factors are involved in the development of psychoses such as schizophrenia (Hunter, 1973; Leonard, 1986; McGuffin et al, 1987). However, social factors are more widely recognised as precipators of episodes of illness, together with the influence of the local environment (Goldstein and Caton, 1983). Brown and his associates have provided one of the most coherent models of this kind for the onset of depression (Brown and Harris, 1978; Brown et al, 1987). They attribute depression to the interaction of 'provoking agents', like bereavement or eviction, with 'vulnerability factors', such as poor social relations and low self-esteem. These ideas have spawned their share of empirical work, for example, on the influence of housing conditions (Freeman, 1984).

Geographical contributions to the causal debates have taken the form of factorial ecologies (Dean and James, 1981; Giggs, 1973; 1986), in which correlations between patterns of illness and attributes of the human and physical environment are searched for. These studies all build on the work of Farris and Dunham (1939), who attributed the concentration of illness rates in Chicago's inner city to the 'social isolation' engendered by such environments. The pronounced clustering observed for schizophrenics has subsequently been attributed to their downward socioeconomic drift, the upward drift of inner-city residents not afflicted by the illness (Miles, 1981), and to ghettoisation (Dear and Moos, 1986), the attraction of cheap rented housing, and health-care facilities.

This variety of interpretation has its roots in the poor understanding of causation, and more applicable results have often been obtained from psychiatric and geographical investigations into illness and type of care. In recent decades the main debate has concerned the pace of 'deinstitutionalisation', which is the process whereby new treatments and policy initiatives have encouraged the transfer of hospital inpatients to community care (Smith and Giggs, 1988). This process is bringing new social problems such as the increasing rates of homelessness observed for the mentally ill in the USA (Morrissey and Gounis, 1988). In addition, the psychiatric services are undergoing organisational upheavals caused by the need to provide alternative forms of community care. For example, in the United Kingdom the Community Psychiatric Nursing Service was introduced to administer long-acting drugs to schizophrenics, but is now playing a wider role in the provision of care (Nutter and Thomas, 1990; Wooff et al, 1988).

The pressure to reorganise psychiatric services has given rise to questions about the general accessibility of patients to the care facilities. It has been known for a long time that service utilisation declines with distance from the facility (Joseph and Phillips, 1984), especially for relatively minor diagnoses such as the neuroses. In addition, the individual referral practices of general practitioners and psychiatric consultants can have an impact on whether a patient is placed in specialised care or not (Joseph, 1979; Joseph and Broeckh, 1981). These findings clearly suggest that alterations to the pattern of service provision should be designed to minimise the geographical isolation of patients. Mathematical programming models offer solutions where new facility locations are determined according to the aggregate travel expenses of patients (Sixsmith, 1988), and Leonardi (1981) has proposed a unifying framework for this subject which is closely related to spatial interaction theory in regional science.

4 Contents
The individual contributions to this volume reflect many of the developments that have just been related. Certain topics, such as the detection of cancer clusters, are given greater coverage to reflect the current balance of research. In contrast, the analysis of health-care delivery systems has been omitted because this topic is the subject of an earlier volume in this series (Clarke, 1984).

The contributions are organised into 4 parts which tackle either specific analytical problems or an issue related to disease incidence and control. Part 1 is primarily concerned with the statistical problems of inferring relationships between point distributions of cases and the location(s) of the hypothesised disease agent. In addition, the emphasis on applications to human cancers provides this section with a subsiduary theme on disease. Part 2 is unambiguously analytical, and examines the problems of both constructing space–time forecasting models and applying their outputs to controlling the spread of disease. Parts 3 and 4 draw together work on disease problems that confront contemporary spatial epidemiology, illustrated by the specific issues raised by the AIDS pandemic, by the provision of care for the mentally ill, and by the sociospatial characteristics of drug abuse. The contents of these main sections are now examined in more detail.

4.1 Statistical analyses of case clustering
This section of the book progresses from the more theoretical to the
applied. In the first 2 papers the evaluation and construction of statistical
tests for identifying case clustering are examined, whereas the authors of
the next 2 are more directly concerned with the inferences that can be
drawn from the detection of apparently significant clusters of cancer cases.

Wartenberg and Greenberg open the section by presenting the results
of simulation experiments where the power of some well-established
tests for space–time clustering is calculated for some hypothetical events.
Power is defined in the statistical sense as the probability that the test
will reject the null hypothesis when this hypothesis is genuinely false.
The tests they choose to study are a cell occupancy statistic, Mantel's
space–time regression (STR), and the spatial autocorrelation coefficients
of Moran and Geary. This selection covers some common types of data
(location of a disease event, distances between all possible pairs of
cases, and distances to a fixed point), and the inclusion of Mantel's STR
provides added generality because other tests, like that of Knox (1963;
1964), are special cases of this regression.

Their findings do not point to a single preferable test on all their
evaluation criteria. However, the results do indicate that tests based on
cross-product statistics (autocorrelation statistics and Mantel's STR)
appear to be more robust. Further application of these procedures to a
wider class of hypothetical events offers the prospect of finding reliable
general detection methods for identifying those case clusters which
warrant further epidemiological investigation.

Diggle et al take a more specific approach to case clustering. Their
problem is to relate the distribution of cancer of the larynx to the location
of a waste incinerator which is the suspected source of carinogens. To
this end they devise a log-likelihood statistic to test the observed intensity
of cases at a given distance from the source, against a background
intensity which is modelled as an inhomogeneous Poisson process. They
choose to estimate the background intensity by using the observed intensity
of lung cancer, which is thought to be unrelated to the outputs of the
incinerator and has a similar age–sex frequency distribution to cancer of
the larynx.

Application of the test to a part of Lancashire indicated a significant
clumping of cases of cancer of the larynx up to 2 km from the incinerator.
However, this result arises from the location of just 5 cases, and the
removal of any one of these cases causes the outcome to be insignificant
at the 5% level. Such fragility is quite a common occurrence in spatial
statistics, where the presence of a few cases in a sparsely populated area
can prove to be critical to the interpretation of the test.

In their paper, Diggle et al discuss the possibility of conducting a more
generalised test where the distribution of disease is compared with
random points in addition to the suspected source. This idea also lies

at the heart of Openshaw's geographical analysis machine (GAM) which, in its various guises as a generalised method of cluster detection, has aroused considerable critical attention in geography, medicine, and the nuclear industry. In the simplest form of the GAM the number of cases falling within a circle of fixed radius is counted and, if this count is significantly in excess of the random expectation, the circle is then plotted on the map. This procedure is repeated for circles of the same radius until the entire study area has been tested. The test continues with larger and larger radii and, on completion, the case clusters are detected as dense patterns of circles ('blobs'). In his paper Openshaw reviews the evolution of the machine as his collaboration with medical practitioners and statisticians has led to refinements and improvements.

Apart from its neat combination of visual simplicity with supercomputer power, interest in the machine has been sustained by the repeated detection of a cluster of childhood leukaemia cases around the Sellafield nuclear reprocessing plant in Cumbria—the implication being that these cases might have been caused by exposure to unsafe levels of radiation. However, Wakeford in his paper succinctly demonstrates that present data and methods are still too inadequate to permit the inference of causation. He argues that factors such as variable efficiency in the registration of cases, poor knowledge of the power of spatial statistics, the sparse incidence of cases of childhood leukaemia in rural areas, and the possible influence of confounding effects not included in the test, all serve to blur the assessment of the radiation risk. These difficulties will ensure that the interpretation of distributions of cancer will remain a dynamic and controversial field of research.

4.2 Forecasting and control

A number of techniques have been devised to forecast the spread and timing of the incidence of infectious diseases. The essential choice is between mathematical and statistical models. A mathematical model is formed from a set of differential equations which describe the transactions which take place between the epidemic populations (susceptibles, infectives, immunes, and so on) in each unit of time. Accurate forecasting depends on the extent to which the differential equations match the behaviour of the disease in question and on the reliable estimation of the transaction rates. The alternative is to identify a purely statistical model that is able to replicate the past incidence of the disease. The parameters of best fit are then used to project the series into the future with the forecast error gradually increasing with each step in time. Many other approaches are possible and most are mixtures of these two basic options (see Cliff et al, 1986).

In the papers in this section the construction and application of some of these models are examined. Cliff and Haggett are particularly concerned with strategies for vaccination and disease control. They examine the way a recurrent epidemic model can be used to test alternative strategies and to estimate critical community size. This last figure is the minimum population necessary for a disease to remain endemic in the community. Using Icelandic data, they identify critical community sizes for measles, rubella, and whooping cough. However, the critical figure for influenza is unstable, probably because, unlike the other diseases, infection with the influenza virus(es) does not confer lifelong immunity. They also make the intriguing suggestion that this instability might imply that there are more drifted subtypes of the influenza virus in circulation than has previously been supposed.

In my paper I am concerned with the ways in which the design of a multiregion model of disease can influence the properties of its forecasts. In particular, the consequences of replacing the standard specification of regionally variable infectivity rates with a single rate are examined in relation to the behaviour of a recurrent epidemic model constructed for Hodgkin's disease. To achieve a single rate specification, ideas from spatial interaction theory are introduced to scale predicted contact totals to the equilibrium incidence of disease in each region.

Simulation experiments with these 2 basic model types reveal a number of effects on the predicted forecasts—the most important finding being a relationship between the time and amplitude of the first epidemic peak and the location of the region which is the source of the simulated epidemic. This time is a constant for a single rate model, irrespective of the source region, but is variable when regional infectivity rates are specified. This relationship between the forecast and the chosen mechanism of spread is symptomatic of the many theoretical problems in multiregion disease modelling that will need to be understood before reliable fore-casting is made possible.

4.3 The AIDS pandemic

The appearance of a new infectious disease in the human population has always provided a source of alarm and uncertainty. Such reactions are most intense during the early stages of the epidemic when the risks to different groups are poorly understood. In both papers in this section, this problem of interpreting the historical spread of AIDS during its first epidemic wave is confronted. Dutt et al examine the composition of US AIDS victims since the disease gained a foothold there in 1981. They chart the relative decline in the importance of male homosexual victims parallelled by the growing importance of intravenous drug misusers. A further consequence of this trend is the increased incidence of AIDS among blacks and new-born children.

Whereas Dutt et al are concerned foremost with the spread of the main agent of AIDS, the HIV-1 virus, Smallman-Raynor and Cliff turn their attention to the newer wave of AIDS due its viral relative HIV-2.

From an extensive survey of the epidemiological literature, they then chart the progress of HIV-2 from its African origins into Europe, in particular to Portugal, and present a composite model for its global distribution. They stress that the early detection of HIV-2 in relation to its associated epidemic offers much greater scope for reconstructing its initial spread than was the case with HIV-1, whose beginnings were obscured by poor-quality data prior to its isolation. Their reconstruction suggests that HIV-2 might infect the at-risk populations in different proportions from those currently observed for HIV-1. For example, female prostitutes are often cited as playing a key role in the spread of HIV-2. The recent origins of the HIV-2 epidemic make enlightened speculation about future progress difficult; however, Smallman-Raynor and Cliff's concluding research agenda points to what is bound to be a challenging field of epidemiological inquiry.

4.4 Mental health and the environment

The papers in the final part address the much more long-standing problem of the influence of the environment on both the care and prevalence of mental disorder. Scobie's central concern is with the role of the general practitioner (GP) as a filter between illness in the community and treatment at a specialised psychiatric agency. She makes use of the records of patients on the Salford Psychiatric Case Register, and manipulates these records to construct incidence rates for a variety of disorders at each practice in the city. These surrogates for referral rates become the dependent variables in a series of multiple regression models which each contain as independent variables the average list size of GPs, the presence of a community psychiatric nurse at the practice, and the social status of the area around the practice.

Her results are decisive, and indicate that average list size is the dominant influence on referral rates. GPs with long lists refer significantly fewer cases of mental illness, and this effect is most pronounced for patients suffering from psychosocial problems such as anxiety disorders and drug dependencies. These results have important policy implications, because the proposed financial incentives for GPs in the United Kingdom are likely to result in longer lists and shorter consultation times.

The final paper, by Giggs, tackles the problems of drug abuse more explicitly. He begins by examining the growth and distribution of drug abuse in the United Kingdom, and discusses the difficulties of interpreting official statistics. It is stressed that the need to control drug abuse has become increasingly important in the 1980s, when the possibility of HIV infection through a shared syringe has added to the health risks already related to addiction. He provides an introduction to a study of illegal drug abuse in Nottingham, in which he uses a multiagency enumeration technique to identify class A drug users. He applies a principal components analysis in combination with multiple regression to demonstrate that strong links exist between levels of drug abuse, poor social and material resources, an inner-city milieu, and some life-cycle and tenure constructs. Analyses of individual drug users reveal high levels of residential mobility and a complication of the relationship between abuse and low socioeconomic status because of factors such as local policies on housing allocation and the location of networks of drug supply.

A feature of the papers in parts 3 and 4 is their extensive reviews of literature, which makes their contents especially useful for researchers who are beginning their studies. Indeed, all the papers are written with a clarity that will appeal to undergraduates taking courses in medical geography or epidemiology. However, the principal objective in this book is to cast new light on some of the contemporary spatial problems that are likely to confront epidemiology throughout the 1990s.

Acknowledgement. I wish to thank the British Academy for assistance.

References
Bailey N J T, 1975 *The Mathematical Theory of Infectious Diseases* (Charles Griffin, London)
Barker D J P, 1982 *Practical Epidemiology* (Churchill Livingstone, Edinburgh)
Barker D J P, Rose R, 1984 *Epidemiology in Medical Practice* (Churchill Livingstone, Edinburgh)
Brown G W, Harris T, 1978 *The Social Origins of Depression* (Tavistock Publications, Andover, Hants)
Brown G W, Bifulco A, Harris T, 1987, "Life events, vulnerability and the onset of depression" *British Journal of Psychiatry* **150** 30 – 42
Burkitt D P, 1969, "Etiology of Burkitt's lymphoma" *Journal of the National Cancer Institute* **42** 19
Carne C A, Weller I V D, Johnson A M, Loveday C, Pearce F, Hawkins A, Smith A, Williams P, Tedder R S, Alder M W, 1987, "Prevalence of antibodies to human immunodeficiency virus, gonorrhoea rates, and changed sexual behaviour in homosexual men in London" *Lancet* **i** 656 – 658
CDSC, 1988, "Communicable disease report 88/01", Communicable Disease Surveillance Centre, Public Health Laboratory Service, 61 Colindale Avenue, London NW9 5HT, England
Clarke M (Ed.), 1984 *London Papers in Regional Science 13: Planning and Analysis in Health Care Systems* (Pion, London)
Cliff A D, Haggett P, Ord J K, 1986 *Spatial Aspects of Influenza Epidemics* (Pion, London)
Cliff A D, Haggett P, Ord J K, Versey G R, 1981 *Spatial Diffusion: An Historical Geography of Epidemics in an Island Community* (Cambridge University Press, Cambridge)
Dean K G, James H D, 1981, "Social factors and admission to psychiatric hospitals: schizophrenia in Plymouth" *Transactions of the Institute of British Geographers: New Series* **6** 39 – 52
Dear M J, Moos A I, 1986, "Structuration theory in urban analysis: 2. Empirical application" *Environment and Planning A* **18** 351 – 373
Doll R, Peto R, 1976, "Mortality in relation to smoking: twenty years of observations on male doctors" *British Medical Journal* series 2, 1525 – 1536
Dubos R, 1959 *Mirage of Health* (Harper and Row, New York)

Dutt A K, Monroe C B, Dutta H M, Prince B, 1987, "Geographical patterns of AIDS in the United States" *Geographical Review* **77** 456–471

Epstein M A, Achong B G, 1979 *The Epstein–Barr Virus* (Springer, New York)

Farris R E L, Dunham H W, 1939 *Mental Disorders in Urban Areas* (University of Chicago Press, Chicago, IL)

Freeman H L (Ed.), 1984 *Mental Health and the Environment* (Churchill Livingstone, Edinburgh)

Giggs J A, 1973, "The distribution of schizophrenics in Nottingham" *Transactions of the Institute of British Geographers* **59** 55–76

Giggs J A, 1986, "Mental disorders and ecological structure in Nottingham" *Social Science and Medicine* **23** 945–961

Gilbert E W, 1958, "Pioneer maps of health and disease in England" *Geographical Journal* **124** 172–183

Goldstein J M, Caton C L M, 1983, "The effects of community environment on chronic psychiatric patients" *Psychological Medicine* **13** 193–199

Good C M, 1986 *Ethnomedical Systems in Africa* (Guildford Press, New York)

Gould P, 1985 *The Geographer at Work* (Routledge, Chapman and Hall, Andover, Hants)

Greenberg M R, 1983 *Urbanization and Cancer Mortality* (Oxford University Press, New York)

Haynes R, 1987 *The Geography of Health Services in Great Britain* (Croom Helm, Andover, Hants)

Howe G M (Ed.), 1977 *A World Geography of Human Disease* (Academic Press, New York)

Hunter R, 1973, "Psychiatry and neurology: psychosyndrome or brain disease?" *Proceedings of the Royal Society of Medicine* **66** 17–22

Hutt M S R, Burkitt D P, 1986 *The Geography of Non-infectious Disease* (Oxford University Press, Oxford)

Illich I, 1975 *Medical Nemesis* (Pantheon Books, New York)

Jones K, Moon G, 1987 *Health, Disease and Society* (Routledge, Chapman and Hall, Andover, Hants)

Joseph A E, 1979, "The referral system as a modifier of distance decay effects in the utilization of mental health services" *Canadian Geographer* **23** 159–169

Joseph A E, Broeckh J L, 1981, "Locational variation in mental health care utilization dependent on diagnosis" *Social Science and Medicine* **15** 395–404

Joseph A E, Phillips D R, 1984 *Accessibility and Utilization: Geographical Perspectives on Health Care Delivery* (Harper and Row, New York)

Knox E G, 1963, "Detection of low intensity epidemicity, application to cleft lip and palate" *British Journal of Preventative and Social Medicine* **17** 121–127

Knox E G, 1964, "Detection of space–time interaction" *Applied Statistician* **13** 25–29

Knox E G, 1986, "A transmission model for AIDS" *European Journal of Epidemiology* **2** 165–177

Leonard K, 1986, "Different causation factors in different forms of schizophrenia" *British Journal of Psychiatry* **149** 1–6

Leonardi G, 1981, "A unifying framework for public facility location problems— part 1: A critical overview and some unsolved problems" *Environment and Planning A* **13** 1001–1028

McGuffin P, Farmer A, Gottesman I, 1987, "Is there really a split in schizophrenia?" *British Journal of Psychiatry* **150** 581–582

McKeown T, 1979 *The Role of Medicine: Dream, Mirage or Nemesis?* (Basil Blackwell, Oxford)

Mangoud A, Hillier V F, Leck I, Thomas R W, 1985, "Space-time interaction in Hodgkin's disease in Greater Manchester" *Journal of Epidemiology and Community Health* **39** 58-62

May J M, 1950, "Medical geography: its methods and objectives" *Geographical Review* **40** 9-41

May J M, 1960 *Disease Ecology* (Hafner Press, New York)

Mayer J D, 1988, "The spatial epidemiology of pandemic influenza in Seattle, 1918-1919" *Geography Research Forum* **8** 90-101

Meade M, Florin J, Gesler W, 1988 *Medical Geography* (Guildford Press, New York)

Miles A, 1981 *The Mentally-ill in Contemporary Society* (Martin Robertson, Oxford)

Morrissey J P, Gounis K, 1988, "Homelessness and mental illness in America: emerging issues in the construction of a social problem", in *Location and Stigma: Contemporary Perspectives on Mental Health and Mental Health Care* Eds C J Smith, J A Giggs (Unwin Hyman, London) pp 285-303

Nutter R D, Thomas R W, 1990, "An analysis of psychiatric patient attributes in Salford using categorical data models" *Social Science and Medicine* **30** 83-94

Openshaw S, 1977, "A geographical solution to scale and aggregation problems in region building, partitioning and spatial modelling" *Transactions of the Institute of British Geographers: New Series* **2** 459-472

Openshaw S, Charlton M, Craft A, 1988, "Searching for leukemia clusters using a geographical analysis machine" *Papers of Regional Science Association* **64** 95-106

Pyle G F, 1979 *Applied Medical Geography* (John Wiley, New York)

Sixsmith A J, 1988, "Locating mental health facilities: a case study", in *Location and Stigma: Contemporary Perspectives on Mental Health and Mental Health Care* Eds C J Smith, J A Giggs (Unwin Hyman, London) pp 175-202

Smallman-Raynor M R, Cliff A D, 1990, "Acquired immune deficiency syndrome (AIDS): literature, geographical origins and global patterns" *Progress in Human Geography* **14**

Smith C J, Giggs J A (Eds), 1988 *Location and Stigma: Contemporary Perspectives on Mental Health and Mental Health Care* (Unwin Hyman, London)

Snow J, 1855 *On the Mode of Transmission of Cholera* (Harvard University Press, Cambridge, MA)

Thomas R W, 1981, "Point pattern analysis", in *Quantitative Geography: A British View* Eds N Wrigley, R J Bennett (Routledge, Chapman and Hall, Andover, Hants) pp 164-176

Thomas R W, 1988, "Stochastic carrier models for the simulation of Hodgkin's disease in a system of regions" *Environment and Planning A* **20** 1575-1601

Weiner I B, Del Gaudio A C, 1976, "Psychopathology in adolescence" *Archives of General Psychiatry* **33** 187-193

Wooff K, Goldberg D P, Fryers T, 1988, "The practice of community psychiatric nursing and mental health social work in Salford: some implications for community care" *British Journal of Psychiatry* **152** 783-792

Part 1

Statistical Analysis of Case Clustering

Space-Time Models for the Detection of Clusters of Disease

D WARTENBERG
University of Medicine and Dentistry of New Jersey, Piscataway, NJ
M GREENBERG
Rutgers University, New Brunswick, NJ

1 Introduction

The investigation by health officials of disease clusters is an activity that is taking on increased importance in government agencies. Although some may argue about its categorisation as a type of epidemiological investigation (Rothman, 1990), few argue about the growing public concern over environmentally caused disease or the political need for a coherent response to inquiries about anomalous disease patterns. Most states in the USA have developed programs for responding to cluster investigation requests (Greenberg and Wartenberg, 1989). These programs parse out requests into those that most likely are unusual occurrences and those that are not. After preliminary investigations and data collection for those situations that appear worrisome, some type of statistical evaluation is made to determine whether or not to pursue an in-depth or full-scale epidemiological investigation. It is the nature of some of those statistical evaluations that we consider in this study.

The evaluations need to be quick, easy to perform and interpret, and responsive to perceived problems. Thus, a variety of methods have been proposed to assess small-sample, rare-disease data. Ideally, these methods should be reliable statistically. Surprisingly, the reliability of such tests have been evaluated only occasionally and most often the tests are applied in response to purported clusters rather than for routine systematic evaluation. Two parameters of particular importance in assessing the reliability of these methods are the sensitivity (statistical power, type 2 errors) and the specificity (type 1 errors). The former is an index of how unusual a pattern must be for a method to detect it. The latter is an index of how likely it is that a pattern will erroneously be found to be unusual.

In this paper, we consider methods for detecting space-time clusters only. Purely spatial and purely temporal clusters will be considered elsewhere. We focus on 2 research questions: (1) "What are the advantages and disadvantages of widely used methods of cluster detection for the discovery of disease patterns that might occur as a result of environmental exposures?" and (2) "Are there cluster detection methods, statistics, or simulation procedures that are so disadvantageous that they can produce misleading results?" We present a typology of cluster investigation methods, and consider a few of these methods in detail and evaluate their statistical properties. We perform a series of simulations to evaluate what types of disease excesses can be detected by specific methods and how large these excesses must be for detection. We show that the nature of the simulation, the null hypothesis, and any alternative hypothesis all have important effects on the results. Consequently, although few practitioners consider the consequences of the methods of simulation and the formulation of the null hypothesis, we suggest that the power and sensitivity of the methods should be an explicit part of the design of the investigation of disease excess.

2 Methods
2.1 Analytic strategy
To organise our work, we have created a typology of methods based on their approach to disease clustering. We hope that our classification will help practitioners choose methods most appropriate to a particular application and enable theoreticians to identify gaps and patterns in methodological development. After separating the methods by the spatiotemporal domain they cover (space, time, or space–time), we use 4 categories to classify the methods.

First, a *data type* is selected. Generally, this is the location of a disease event, the distance between all pairs of events, the nearest-neighbor distance between events, or the distance to a fixed point.

Second, we select a *transformation type*. We may wish to use ranks to protect against outlier data values or to take the inverse of the distances to increase the relative importance of close pairs and decrease the importance of distant pairs. (In taking inverses, one must first add a constant to the distances to allow for taking the inverse of near zero distances.) Or, we may use some other type of transformation, or none at all. In some methods transformations are used to accommodate variation among confounding variables.

Third, we select a *summary statistic* to characterise our data. Examples include counts per cell (for cell occupancy methods), mean distances (for some point pattern methods), and the correlation between spatial and temporal distances (for Mantel's space–time method).

Fourth, we use a method to generate the *reference distribution* with which to compare the observed statistic. This reference distribution may be specified a priori (as in the 'ridit' approach—for example, see Pinkel et al, 1963), or may be derived analytically or via permutational simulation. In some methods, the reference distribution is used to accommodate information on confounding variables.

The first method we use in this study is Ederer, Myers, and Mantel's (1964) (EMM) which is a type of cell occupancy approach. The study area is divided into a series of subregions and the total time of observation is split into a number of time periods. For each geographic subregion considered, the maximum number of events in any specified time period is tabulated and the sum of these maximum values over time within a subregion are compared with a value derived analytically. According to our typology, the counts are used in the method as a data type; the data are not transformed; the summary statistic is the maximum number of events in any time period summed over all subregions; and the reference distribution is derived analytically.

The second method we use is Mantel's (1967) space-time regression (STR) in which spatial interevent distances are correlated with temporal interevent distances. The data type is interevent distances; the data are not transformed, or they are inverse or inverse-squared transformed; the summary statistic is the correlation coefficient; and the distribution is analytically derived. In this paper, we report results obtained by using the inverse distance transformation with a constant of 0.1.

The third and fourth methods we use are spatial autocorrelation statistics: Moran's 'I' method (MI) and Geary's 'c' method (Gc) (Cliff and Ord, 1981). Although generally these indices are used to look only at the spatial pattern of a particular variate, we use them to look for spatiotemporal patterns by evaluating the spatial autocorrelation of the time of occurrence of disease events. We use 2 data types: spatial interevent distance and time of occurrence. We transform the spatial distance by taking the inverse square and do not transform the temporal data. The summary statistic is a scaled cross-product (Hubert, 1987), a correlation coefficient. The reference distribution is derived analytically. This Gc method is identical to the STR method if the spatial distance matrix in the STR is given an inverse square transformation and the temporal distance matrix is given a square transformation.

We selected the first 2 methods for evaluation because of their widespread citation in the literature. They represent 2 fundamentally different approaches to the detection of clusters. The EMM method is a type of cell occupancy approach in which the study region is divided into a series of time-space subregions and in which it is evaluated whether the distribution of cases in these subregions is unusual. Others (for example, Grimson, 1979; Pinkel and Nefzger, 1959) have suggested analogous methods but those methods tend to be used less often. The STR method is one of many that compare interevent distances in space and time (for example, Cruickshank, 1947; Grimson et al, 1981; Knox, 1963). Again, it seems to be the most popular choice by practitioners for this type of method. We chose the autocorrelation statistics because of their broad utility, the more rigorous statistical study that they have been subjected to, and the appearance of these methods in the epidemiological literature (for example, Clapp et al, 1989; Cook and Pocock, 1983; Raubertas, 1988; Tango, 1984).

2.2 Simulation strategy

In this study 2 types of simulation are used. The first is a model of disease process that produces a hypothetical pattern. That is, cases of disease, or events, are distributed at random in space and time according to a specified rule. Different rules can be used to simulate different types of disease processes. For example, one subregion may be hypothesised to be at higher risk. In the simulation, this subregion would get proportionally more cases than the rest of the study area, that is, it would have a greater density of cases. The second type of simulation is a randomisation or permutation of the hypothetical pattern. This simulation is used to evaluate statistical significance of the hypothetical pattern. If the hypothetical pattern gives a statistic that is larger (or smaller) than most of the values of the statistic calculated for the permuted patterns, it is found to be statistically significant. In general, in this paper the word *simulation* will be used to denote the second approach.

Developing a strategy for generating and evaluating patterns showing the absence or presence of disease has turned out to be more complex than we had anticipated. In our previous work (Wartenberg and Greenberg, 1989), we used a standard strategy for evaluating the EMM and STR methods. We simulated 2 simple patterns of disease and evaluated their statistical significance by using the analytic approximations provided by the authors who developed the methods. We found that both the EMM and the STR had low power; that is, they produced an unusually large number of false negatives under our 2 models of clustering. Further, their sensitivity varied by cluster type. These results caused us to reconsider our evaluation procedure.

Our strategy had been to generate various cluster patterns and to test the methods on these patterns. For generated data sets that have a random distribution of cases, or no clustering, we want to determine how often a statistically significant cluster is detected—in other words, the probability of false positives (or type 1 or α errors); that is, statistically significant results are obtained even though there is no consistent, underlying pattern to the data or the generating process. Statistically, the false positive rate is the frequency with which we reject the null hypothesis even though it is true. For generated data sets that have nonrandom (clinal or hot-spot) patterns, we want to determine how often a statistically significant result is not detected—in other words, the probability of false negatives (or type 2 or β errors); that is, results are obtained that fail to detect a cluster even though one exists. Statistically, the false negative rate is the frequency with which we fail to reject the null hypothesis even though it is false. The power is calculated as 1.0 minus the false negative rate (that is, the frequency with which we reject the null hypothesis when it is false).

We conducted our initial evaluation with use of the first 2 distributional moments [derived by Mantel (1967) for the STR method, and by Ederer et al (1964) and Mantel et al (1976) for the EMM method], assuming the standardised statistic to be approximately normal. One observation we made in a previous study (Wartenberg and Greenberg, 1989) was that the equation for the approximation of the analytic distribution of the EMM method provided by Stark and Mantel (1967) and Mantel et al (1976) was not sufficiently accurate for use in the evaluation of simulations. Its use gave a large number of false positives that increased with increasing numbers of cases. However, under the null model, using the tabulated results of Mantel et al (1976), we achieved expected error rates.

Klauber (1971), Siemiatycki (1978), Mielke (1978), Dietz (1983), and Manly (1986) have pointed out the inadequacy of the approximation for the STR method. Our results (Wartenberg and Greenberg, 1989) were consistent with these findings. Siemiatycki (1978) derived the third and fourth moments of this method and compared the results with a Pearson probability distribution. Finding the first 4 moments and fitting them to a Pearson curve, although simpler computationally than permutational simulation, still is complex. We chose to omit this method as we regarded it as being too difficult for the untrained investigator and numerically inferior to permutational simulation (discussed below) for the sophisticated user.

In general, investigators recommend using simulation or randomisation methods when possible. Klauber (1971) presented 2 randomisation approaches for evaluating the STR structure. In one it is assumed that one set of distances (for example, all event locations) are fixed and the other set of distances (for example, all event times) are random. The second approach assumes that both sets of distances (for example, event locations and times) are random. Both false positive and false negative results were observed, and Klauber cautions users to beware of the high sensitivity of this method to clusters of just a few points. Using reciprocal distances, he found that significant space-time clustering was detected even when none actually existed. Siemiatycki (1978) performed simulations on a real data set by permuting the times of disease occurrence and holding the disease locations constant. He found that the power of the analytic approximation was poorer than his more complicated approximation, but acknowledges the superiority of permutational methods if sufficient computing resources are available.

Dietz (1983) generated data by perturbing a set of 2-dimensional, uniformly distributed coordinates twice independently to generate 2 sets of distances. The perturbation was an addition to each variable of a random value drawn from a uniform random distribution $(-u, u)$. The range of the random error values controlled the degree of association. She then assumed one set of distances was fixed, and she permuted the other. Similarly, Manly (1986), in a series of simulations, evaluated distances calculated from 2-coordinate and 3-coordinate, uniformly distributed, random data. The 3-coordinate data (x_i, y_i, z_i) share the same 2-coordinate values as the 2-coordinate data (x_i, y_i). He also varied the range of the third coordinate to control the level of association. He fixed one distance matrix but regenerated the other repeatedly. Both of these researchers evaluated the power of the statistics, but their formulations cannot be directly related to current study owing to different parameterisations of association.

Chen et al (1984) studied the power of the EMM and STR methods for detecting simulated patterns of an infectious disease (Hodgkin's disease). Because of the aetiology of the disease studied, the patterns were composed of many small clusters distributed throughout the data field in contrast to the more spatially coherent patterns we investigate. Overall, they found the methods to be weak and suggest that failure to detect clusters in some situations may be due to the low power of a statistical technique rather than the absence of pattern.

Many others have evaluated cluster statistics by assessing pattern in real data sets. Although useful for studying disease, these evaluations are not directly comparable with one another owing to the idiosyncrasies of specific diseases and observations. In our experiment, we generate patterns of interest and determine the sensitivity and specificity of the cluster detection methods on these patterns. By applying the methods to patterns for which we know the underlying characteristics, we hope to gain insight into making inferences with real data sets for which we do not know the underlying pattern or the process generating it. The patterns we consider are: (a) random distribution of cases; (b) nonrandom clinal distribution of cases (gradually increasing relative risk; see figure 1); (c) nonrandom hot spots of cases (regions of high relative risk; see figure 1).

We report statistical significance results for these patterns by comparing the patterned data with: (1) an analytic approximation of the distribution of the statistic for each method; (2) statistics simulated from data with random spatial coordinates with random times of occurrence; and (3) statistics simulated from data with fixed, observed spatial coordinates and permuted, observed times of occurrence. We did not evaluate simulations with fixed spatial coordinates and random times of occurrence. The analytic approximations are given in Ederer et al (1964), Mantel (1967), and Mantel et al (1976). We report results for nominal, 2-tailed, 5% error rates. Evaluations of the randomised simulation were derived by repeatedly (1000 times) generating a specified number of cases (ranging from 5 to 50) in our time–space domain, finding in each tail of the distribution that point at which only 2.5% of the simulations were more extreme for each sample size, and applying them to another set of 1000 simulations. Evaluations of the permutation simulation were derived by repeatedly (50 times) generating a specified number of cases (ranging from 5 to 50) in our time–space domain and permuting the times of occurrence 50 times for the same set of spatial locations (each number is the result of 2500 simulations).

We conducted these experiments for each of the 3 scenarios. First, for the null case, we assumed that all locations have equal risk of event occurrence and we distributed cases at random. That is, we assigned random values (uniform [0, 1]) to geographic (x, y) and temporal (t) coordinates for each case. A plot of the relative risk (RR) across the surface is shown as the solid curve in figure 1 (RR equal to 1). This curve represents a transect from the origin of our time–space domain to the opposite corner [that is, from $(0, 0, 0)$ to $(1, 1, 1)$]. We subdivided the transect into 20 segments and calculated the average number of cases observed in each segment under this scenario. We divided this number by the number of cases observed in the last cell $(1, 1, 1)$ and plotted the result.

Similarly, we generated surfaces for the 2 types of clusters. The clinal surface represents a gradual change in the risk of event occurrence. One can imagine the cline as a pollution gradient from a point source. Through the processes of advection and diffusion, the concentration falls off as the distance from the point source increases. To derive this surface, we generated random coordinates as above and then raised them to a specified power, in this case to the power 3. By raising the coordinates to a power, we increased the likelihood that events would occur near the origin. The risk surface is smooth and nonlinear, with the magnitude of the power coefficient influencing the steepness of the cline. The relative risk of the clinal surface is shown in figure 1 by the

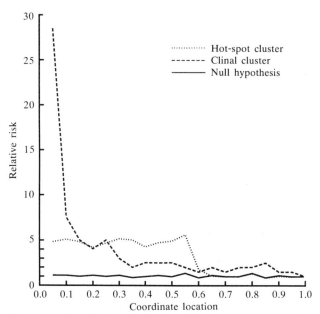

Figure 1. The simulated relative risk along a transect: the simulated relative risk (the ordinate) versus location (the abscissa) along a transect from the origin $(0, 0, 0)$ to the opposite corner $(1, 1, 1)$ is plotted for three different scenarios.

dashed curve, with curvilinearly decreasing relative risk. Under the null hypothesis, an event can occur anywhere in the space–time domain with equal probability. If coordinates are raised to the power 3, 50% of the events, on average, should occur along the first 12.5% of each axis, and over 90% of the events should occur along the first 75% of each axis.

The hot-spot model is a situation in which 1 subregion of the study area has a constant and greater risk than the rest of the study area. An example of a real situation in which such a data pattern is generated is a comparison of individuals receiving contaminated drinking water with those who drink from an uncontaminated source. Individuals within each region incur similar risks but there is a difference between the risks for the 2 regions. To generate this surface, we assign additional cases to the region of elevated relative risk. In this study, the high-risk region includes the origin of our space and represents 20% of the total time–space volume. That is, all points within 0.585 units $(0.20^{1/3})$ of the origin along the x, y, and t axes are in the hot spot and have an elevated relative risk. All other points have a relative risk of 1. The curve denoted by the dotted curve in figure 1 depicts the results of this hot-spot model, showing an increased relative risk of 5 for the first 11 segments and a relative risk of 1 thereafter.

We note that models for the 2 types of patterns we used in this study are simplistic. In these models, simple, isotropic structure in the absence of confounders and edge effects is assumed. Additional models could be developed to include these effects, to consider situations in which the risk is nonuniform over space, time, or population subunit and which have more similarity to the aetiology of a known disease. However, for this study we chose to investigate the simplest hypothesis we could construct. Only if the methods were useful in this simplest of situations would it be useful to consider more complicated scenarios.

In summary, we use 3 patterns in our study. One is random, one clinal, and one is a hot spot. All are shown in figure 1. We also use 3 evaluation strategies. One is based on the analytic approximations of each method, one is based on a set of simulations of null patterns, and one is based on the permuting of the observed time of event occurrence.

3 Results
Results of the simulations described above are presented in figures 2–4. Figure 2 shows false positive rates for all 4 methods in all 3 evaluation procedures. The analytic approximations illustrated in figure 2(a) show that the false positive rates for all methods are close to the expected values but somewhat biased. That is, STR and EMM gave disproportionately more upper-tail false positives, whereas both autocorrelation indices gave disproportionately more lower-tail false positives. Both significance simulation strategies remove this bias problem [see figure 2(b) and 2(c)].

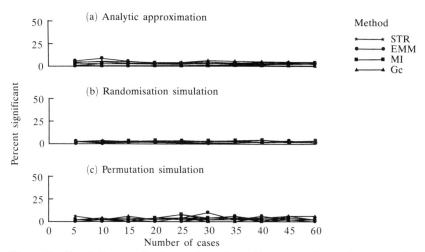

Figure 2. Simulation results for random data. Data were drawn from a random, uniform distribution $(0, 1)$ on each axis. The percentage of simulations that gave significant results (the ordinate) is plotted versus the number of cases in the simulation (the abscissa).

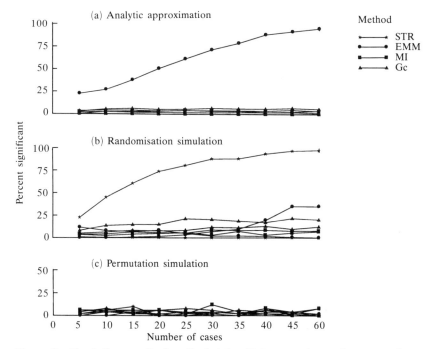

Figure 3. Simulation results for clinal data. Data were drawn from a random, uniform distribution $(0, 1)$ on each axis and cubed to simulate a cline. The percentage of simulations that gave significant results (the ordinate) is plotted versus the number of cases in the simulation (the abscissa).

[We note again, for emphasis, that the equations used for the analytic approximation of the EMM method (Mantel et al, 1976; Stark and Mantel, 1967) are inaccurate for single data sets or simulations and we strongly recommend against their use in these situations.]

Figure 3 shows results from the clinal model for disease occurrence. Under the analytic approximation, only the EMM method detects pattern and it does so with increasing power as the number of cases increases [figure 3(a)]. In the randomisation simulation, the STR method is moderately sensitive to the pattern, with sensitivity increasing as the number of cases increases [figure 3(b)]. Gc shows low sensitivity, detecting a significant pattern 10%–20% of the time, and the EMM method shows increasing sensitivity with the number of cases, beginning at about 30, increasing to about 30% significance at 50 cases. In the permutation simulation none of the methods shows any sensitivity to the patterns [figure 3(c)].

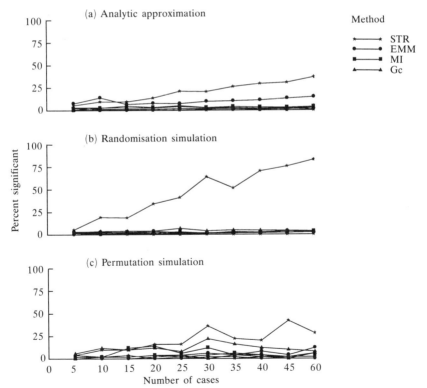

Figure 4. Simulation results for hot-spot data. Data were drawn from a random, uniform distribution (0, 1) on each axis and from a random, uniform distribution (0, 0.585) on each axis to simulate a hot spot (see text). The percentage of simulations that gave significant results (the ordinate) is plotted versus the number of cases in the simulation (the abscissa).

Figure 4 shows results for the hot-spot model. Under the analytic approximation, the STR and EMM methods show weak but increasing power with increasing number of cases [figure 4(a)]. In the randomisation simulation, the STR method again shows substantial sensitivity to the pattern with the magnitude of the sensitivity increasing with increasing numbers of cases [figure 4(b)]. In the permutation simulation the STR shows some weak but consistent sensitivity to the pattern (up to about 30% power), and Gc shows consistent but weaker power (up to about 10% power) [figure 4(c)].

4 Discussion

The simulations performed for this study extend results from our previous work (Wartenberg and Greenberg, 1989) in three ways: (1) they are numerically more extensive; (2) they include 2 additional indices of space-time clustering; and (3) they utilise 2 simulation strategies for significance testing in addition to the analytic approximations used previously. In general, results were consistent with the previous study, were more stable given the greater number of iterations, and have given us additional insight in interpretation. We discuss these observations in terms of models of disease process, detection method tuning, and simulation strategy.

4.1 Models of the disease process

Our main aim in this paper is to compare the sensitivity of some cluster detection methods with particular patterns of disease outcomes. The use of artificially simulated data rather than actual case studies is appropriate for a number of reasons. It allows us to specify particular parameters of the disease process, as we understand it, and determine how their variability influences the power of the methods. It allows us to compare the sensitivity of the detection methods across different types of disease processes. And later, when analysing real data, it allows us to speculate about the type of process that may have given rise to a particular observation by comparison with simulated results and thus to develop hypotheses about observed disease aetiologies. Last, it removes from consideration any idiosyncrasies of true, observed data, such as non-uniform risk surfaces resulting from nonuniform distributions of age, sex, and race.

A wide variety of models which corresponded to different processes could be developed to provide different types of spatiotemporal structure. The principal type of disease we seek to study is that caused by environmental exposures. Most other investigations have evaluated infectious disease patterns or other patterns that do not correspond to our hypotheses for environmental disease. For example, Dietz (1983) and Manly (1986) used a model to induce structure in their data for nonhealth-based application of these same methods. They began with 2

sets of points at identical locations and displaced one set from their
starting locations by moving them from a 2-dimensional plane into a
3-dimensional space (that is, by adding a third coordinte). Thus, they
started with identical configurations and perturbed the data by increasing
amounts. Although this model, which they used to test the similarity of
2 measures of distance on the same set of objects, makes sense in the
context in which they used it, it has little bearing on disease aetiology.
Other researchers (for example, Chen et al, 1984) simulate infectious
disease patterns. These simulations, too, give rise to many small clusters
occurring randomly across the data field. These patterns, however, do
not seem appropriate for environmentally induced disease. It seems
more reasonable to consider regions of elevated risk (the hot-spot model)
or trends of risk from a point source (the clinal model). This subtle
distinction in data generation gave rise to some of the differences in
analytic results.

4.2 Tuning detection methods to a particular hypothesis

Modifications can be made in the cluster detection methods to enhance
their performance. These modifications can be designed for generic
enhancement, such as by using reciprocal distance to emphasise short rather
than long distances, or they can be designed to test specific hypotheses,
such as by calculating distance as lateral distance rather than Euclidean
distance from a polluted stream. Summary statistics can be assessed as
deviations from means, variances, or other measures of pattern, depending
on the hypothesised situation. These modifications can tune a particular
analysis to be most sensitive to a specific type of pattern. The consequence
of this increased sensitivity, of course, is that one loses power against
other types of pattern.

Distance transformation is the modification that has been used most
often by investigators with the STR method. Klauber (1971) used
reciprocal transformations of distance and observed that, with the STR
method, significant clusters were found when none existed and that
transforming the distance data into a binary classification rather than
using the interval data exacerbated the problem. Glass et al (1971), using
reciprocal distances, found that decreasing the size of the additive
constants (used to accommodate the taking of inverses of trivially small
distances) did increase the standard deviates derived from Mantel's
(1967) analytic approximation, often interpreted as showing greater
sensitivity. But, Siemiatycki (1978) found that reciprocal transformations
of distance led to many false positives with Mantel's (1967) analytic
approximation. He rectified this by using his own, more complicated
analytic expression for significance evaluations. He also found that
squaring the inverse distances or changing the additive constants (used
to accommodate the taking of inverses of trivially small distances) did
not affect the result when he used his approximation but did affect the

result when he used Mantel's approximation. Overall, inverse distance transformation seems worthwhile. Our simulations with untransformed distances (not shown) showed virtually no power against the clinal and hot-spot alternatives. The use of reciprocal distances with an additive constant of 0.1 (figures 2-4) was noticeably better for the STR method.

One also can view these modifications as different summary statistics designed to test for particular types of pattern. For example, STR, MI and Gc are specific formulations of the general cross-product statistic or correlations (Hubert, 1987). In STR, the spatial and temporal distances are compared directly. MI uses a set of values defined in this paper as inverse spatial distances and another defined as the product of the temporal deviations from the mean time of occurrences for one event multiplied by the corresponding value for the other event. Gc uses the same spatial distances and the square of the difference between times of occurrence of events for each set of distances. Generally, these coefficients are thought of as different qualitatively, although algorithmically if one uses different formulae to calculate the distances, one can use the same cross-product statistic to evaluate the data.

Many additional modifications are possible. One can build in anisotropic sensitivity with particular angular weighting functions. Or, one can weight distances by confounder scores, such as personal risk.

4.3 Simulation strategies

To judge the effectiveness of the simulation strategies, we compared the power of the methods under both models of disease. Only the STR method showed consistent, substantial power against the alternatives tested. The most effective strategy for significance testing was the randomisation simulation. This result was surprising to us. As various authors had found the analytic approximations to be inadequate (Chen et al, 1984; Dietz, 1983; Klauber, 1971; Manly, 1986; Mielke, 1978; Siemiatycki, 1978), their poor performance was not surprising. However, the poor performance of the permutation simulation in detecting space-time clusters was not expected and caused us to look into this problem in more detail.

For the clinal pattern, the permutation simulation was not effective. Upon review of the data, we noticed that the permuted data were similar in structure to the original data. That is, even after permutation, most of the events were clustered near the origin. This is due, in part, to the fact that the data had been transformed prior to permutation and that only large-scale and no small-scale structure had been induced in the data. Permutation of a set of numbers in which most of the observations are near the origin will result in a different set of numbers, most of which are still near the origin. Consider the example shown in table 1. The first column shows the coordinates (x, y, t) of 5 points drawn from a random uniform distribution. The second column shows these same points after their coordinates are cubed, as in the clinal model. The third and fourth columns show 2 random permutations of these cubed values. The integer values show the grid coordinates for the 5-cell × 5-cell × 5-cell analysis of the EMM method. Even though the data have been randomly permuted, the majority of events in each column occur near the origin. The randomisation simulation for the clinal data, in contrast, distributes cases uniformly and the cluster detection methods show greater sensitivity to the cline. Thus, patterns picked up by the randomisation simulation were not detected by the permutation simulation because the values which were permuted were not a random sample but retained some of the properties of the original data. Even after permutation, there was a preponderance of events near the origin. The nonuniform distribution of cases precludes inferential evaluation with use of permutational simulation. In other words, in the permutational simulation the data are conditional on the distribution of observed values whereas in the randomisation simulation they are not. This conditioning apparently reduces the power of the statistic.

A similar observation can be made for the insensitivity of the permutation process to hot-spot patterns. Most of the cases occur in the hot spot. Consequently, even if the hot spot represents only 20% of the total space–time volume, the hot-spot region dominates the analysis. That is, because the small-scale structure within the hot spot is random, the methods fail to detect the effects of permuting the times of the event occurrences because there are still excess cases within the hot spot with random small-scale structure. Consider the example shown in

Table 1. Simulation of a clinal cluster. The first column contains event coordinates for 5 occurrences drawn from a random, uniform distribution (0, 1). To induce clinal structure in these data, each coordinate is cubed and the resulting coordinates and grid assignments are given in the second column. The next two columns contain coordinates and grid assignments for 5 data points after they have been randomly permuted.

Event	Random data (x, y, t)	Clinal data	Permutation 1	Permutation 2
1	(0.05, 0.24, 0.92)	(0.00, 0.01, 0.79) (1, 1, 4)	(0.00, 0.01, 0.43) (1, 1, 3)	(0.00, 0.01, 0.01) (1, 1, 1)
2	(0.96, 0.53, 0.76)	(0.89, 0.15, 0.43) (5, 1, 3)	(0.89, 0.15, 0.03) (5, 1, 1)	(0.89, 0.15, 0.79) (5, 1,4)
3	(0.90, 0.62, 0.09)	(0.73, 0.24, 0.00) (4, 2, 1)	(0.73, 0.24, 0.00) (4, 2, 1)	(0.73, 0.24, 0.00) (4, 2, 1)
4	(0.13, 0.55, 0.32)	(0.00, 0.16, 0.03) (1, 1, 1)	(0.00, 0.16, 0.01) (1, 1, 1)	(0.00, 0.16, 0.03) (1, 1, 1)
5	(0.47, 0.55, 0.21)	(0.10, 0.16, 0.01) (1, 1, 1)	(0.10, 0.16, 0.79) (1, 1, 4)	(0.10, 0.16, 0.43) (1, 1, 3)

table 2. The first 5 events are taken from a random uniform distribution. The next 3 events are forced to occur in the hot spot. Permutation of these events results in the cell closest to the origin, $(1, 1, 1)$, having the most events. Permutation of only the time coordinate disrupted the small-scale time–space interactions seen in the original data but established some similar interactions. Again, this observation is a consequence of the disease model used to generate the data and is discussed below. Use of inverse transformed distances for the STR statistic emphasised the smallest distances and increased the ability to detect this pattern.

One way to envision these 2 ways of evaluating statistical significance is that the permutation approach is conditional on the time values used in the disease pattern simulation whereas the randomisation approach is unconditional. That is, the permutational approach simply rearranges values, and if these values are predominantly small all rearrangements will continue to contain small numbers. The randomisation, on the other hand, draws times of occurrence from a random, uniform distribution irrespective of the pattern used. Conditional models are more restrictive and thus may have less statistical power.

As Chen et al (1984), Dietz (1983), and Manly (1986) began with small-scale structure, permutational methods which disrupt this structure are useful in evaluating the statistical significance of their observations.

Table 2. Simulation of a hot-spot cluster. The first column contains event coordinates for 5 occurrences drawn from a random, uniform $(0, 1)$ distribution. To induce the hot-spot structure in these data, 3 additional points have been drawn at random from the defined hot spot [a random, uniform distribution $(0, 0.585)$ for each coordinate axis]. The grid assignments for the EMM method are shown below each set of coordinates. The last 2 columns contain coordinates and grid assignments for 5 data points after they have been randomly permuted.

Event	Hot spot	Permutation 1	Permutation 2
1	(0.94, 0.01, 0.58)	(0.94, 0.01, 0.18)	(0.94, 0.01, 0.19)
	(5, 1, 3)	(5, 1, 1)	(5, 1, 1)
2	(0.06, 0.61, 0.38)	(0.06, 0.61, 0.38)	(0.06, 0.61, 0.52)
	(1, 4, 2)	(1, 4, 2)	(1, 4, 3)
3	(0.94, 0.15, 0.21)	(0.94, 0.15, 0.09)	(0.94, 0.15, 0.21)
	(5, 1, 2)	(5, 1, 1)	(5, 1, 2)
4	(0.53, 0.60, 0.09)	(0.53, 0.60, 0.21)	(0.53, 0.60, 0.38)
	(3, 3, 1)	(3, 3, 2)	(3, 3, 2)
5	(0.79, 0.17, 0.74)	(0.79, 0.17, 0.74)	(0.79, 0.17, 0.09)
	(4, 1, 4)	(4, 1, 4)	(4, 1, 1)
6	(0.15, 0.38, 0.18)	(0.15, 0.38, 0.52)	(0.15, 0.38, 0.74)
	(1, 2, 1)	(1, 2, 3)	(1, 2, 4)
7	(0.45, 0.13, 0.19)	(0.45, 0.13, 0.58)	(0.45, 0.13, 0.18)
	(3, 1, 1)	(3, 1, 3)	(3, 1, 1)
8	(0.09, 0.22, 0.52)	(0.09, 0.22, 0.19)	(0.09, 0.22, 0.58)
	(1, 2, 3)	(1, 2, 1)	(1, 2, 3)

Our models induce only broad-scale structure and, in general, induce much weaker patterns. Thus, the permutational methods that Dietz (1983) and Manly (1986) used were not as useful for our study. Without use of a reciprocal transformation of distance, the method showed no power to detect either the clinal or the hot-spot pattern. Even with reciprocal transformations, the randomisation method still is far superior. The randomisation method will work and has superior power for models such as those of Dietz (1983) and Manly (1986) as well as ours, and thus is preferable.

One reason that it is important to consider both of these simulation methods is that although the randomisation method shows greater power in real-world situations, one often does not have sufficient information to perform a randomisation. To do so, one needs baseline risk information about all the individuals in the study to simulate the null or expected distribution. Without such information, one is constrained to using the conditional or permutational approach. Here one uses the distribution of cases as observed and one rearranges their sequence only.

Given the limited utility of permutational simulation for significance testing in this case, the successful use of such an approach to detect disease clusters in other circumstances may seem surprising (for example, Klauber, 1971). However, in these cases, we believe the methods are detecting situations of particularly high risk (small number of background cases) or small clusters within a much larger data field. In our simulations, if we had expanded our data field of background risk and thus the overall number of cases detected, we likely would have been able to use the permutational simulation approach. Or, similarly, if we had increased the relative risk we would have detected unusual patterns. However, as most of the data sets that practitioners must evaluate consist of at most a few dozen cases, and as most environmental risks are thought to be less than 5-fold, we saw our modeling approach as being the most relevant to the real world. These results suggest that many evaluations of cluster data based on permuting the data are too conservative and may have failed to detect truly anomalous situations for purely statistical reasons.

5 Conclusions

The results of our study suggest that methods used for disease cluster investigation are problematic. Simulation must be used to evaluate significance levels or results will be uninterpretable. But one must be sure that the results are compared with an appropriate null model, which may not be provided by permutational simulation. Randomisation appears robust to the choice of a pattern generating model. Last, the cross-product statistic (of which STR, MI, and Gc are special cases, as are a number of other methods) seems most useful and robust. Further investigations are necessary to evaluate the appropriate data transformations to optimise use of the cross-product statistic, but inverse-power transformations seem satisfactory. Simulations of a more extensive nature are needed to validate these conclusions and additional methodological work is needed to provide means for confounder adjustments. Finally, one must pay careful attention to the hypothesis under investigation and make sure that the cluster statistic is sensitive to the particular pattern one wishes to detect.

Acknowledgements. This work was funded by and undertaken in a cooperative agreement with the New Jersey Department of Health.

References

Chen R, Mantel N, Klingberg M A, 1984, "A study of three techniques for time–space clustering in Hodgkin's disease" *Statistics in Medicine* **3** 173–184

Clapp R, Wartenberg D, Cupples L A, 1989, "Statistical methods for analyzing cancer clusters", paper presented at the National Conference on Clustering of Health Events, Atlanta, February; copy available from D Wartenberg

Cliff A D, Ord J K, 1981 *Spatial Processes: Models and Applications* (Pion, London)

Cook D G, Pocock S J, 1983, "Multiple regression in geographic mortality studies with spatially correlated errors" *Biometrics* **39** 361–371

Cruickshank D B, 1947, "Regional influence in cancer" *British Journal of Cancer* **1** 109–128

Dietz E J, 1983, "Permutation tests for association between two distance matrices" *Systematic Zoology* **32** 21–26

Ederer F, Myers M H, Mantel N, 1964, "A statistical problem in space and time: do leukemia cases come in clusters?" *Biometrics* **20** 626–638

Glass A G, Mantel N, Gunz F W, Spears G F S, 1971, "Time–space clustering of childhood leukemia in New Zealand" *Journal of the National Cancer Institute* **47** 329–336

Greenberg M, Wartenberg D, 1989, "State government responses to community requests for cancer cluster investigations: an analysis of alternative process", a report submitted to the New Jersey Department of Health, November 1989; copy available from authors

Grimson R C, 1979, "The clustering of disease" *Mathematical Biosciences* **20** 626–638

Grimson R C, Wang K C, Johnson P W C, 1981, "Searching for hierarchical clusters of disease: spatial patterns of sudden infant death syndrome" *Social Sciences and Medicine* **15D** 287–293

Hubert L J, 1987 *Assignment Methods in Combinatorial Data Analysis* (Marcel Dekker, New York)

Klauber M R, 1971, "Two-sample randomization tests for space–time clustering" *Biometrics* **27** 129–142

Knox G, 1963, "Detection of low intensity epidemicity: application to cleft lip and palate" *British Journal of Preventive and Social Medicine* **17** 121–127

Manly B F J, 1986, "Randomization and regression methods for testing for associations with geographical, environmental and biological distances between populations" *Research in Population Ecology* **28** 201–218

Mantel N, 1967, "The detection of disease clustering and a generalized regression approach" *Cancer Research* **27** 209–220

Mantel N, Kryscio R J, Myers M H, 1976, "Tables and formulas for extended use of the Ederer–Myers–Mantel disease-clustering procedure" *American Journal of Epidemiology* **104** 576–584

Mielke P W, 1978, "Clarification and appropriate inferences for Mantel and Valand's nonparametric multivariate analysis technique" *Biometrics* **34** 277–282

Pinkel D, Nefzger D, 1959, "Some epidemiological features of childhood leukemia in the Buffalo, N.Y. area" *Cancer* **12** 351–357

Pinkel D, Dowd J E, Bross I D J, 1963, "Some epidemiological features of malignant solid tumors of children in Buffalo, N.Y. area" *Cancer* **16** 28–33

Raubertas R F, 1988, "Spatial and temporal analysis of disease occurrence for detection of clusters" *Biometrics* **44** 1121–1129

Rothman K J, 1990, "A sobering start for the cluster busters conference", forthcoming in *American Journal of Epidemiology*

Siemiatycki J, 1978, "Mantel's space–time clustering statistic: computing higher moments and a comparison of various data transforms" *Journal of Statistical Computation and Simulation* **7** 13–31

Stark C R, Mantel N, 1967, "Lack of seasonal or temporal–spatial clustering of Down's syndrome births in Michigan" *American Journal of Epidemiology* **86** 199–213

Tango T, 1984, "The detection of disease clustering in time" *Biometrics* **40** 15–26

Wartenberg D, Greenberg M, 1989, "Detecting disease clusters: the importance of statistical power", paper presented at the National Conference on Clustering of Health Events, Atlanta, February: copy available from D Wartenberg (in press *American Journal of Epidemiology*)

Modelling the Prevalence of Cancer of the Larynx in Part of Lancashire: A New Methodology for Spatial Epidemiology

P J DIGGLE, A C GATRELL, A A LOVETT
Lancaster University

1 Introduction

The availability of high-quality epidemiological data in Britain, notably from cancer registries, coupled with the advent of geographical information systems, has given fresh impetus to research into disease clustering. Such data are frequently available at a very fine level of spatial resolution, permitting the description and analysis of diseases in very localised regions. There is now a growing literature, with contributions from geographers, statisticians, and epidemiologists, on methods for detecting 'clusters' of such diseases (Elliot, 1988), and such methodologies are outlined briefly below. In this paper we follow in this tradition, but seek to go beyond the recognition of a cluster by formulating a model of disease prevalence that allows for the explicit testing of a hypothesised environmental association.

We may take a disease cluster to be "any localised spatial aggregation of cases" (Alexander et al, 1988, page 23), though we should of course recognise that diseases may be clustered in time and in space – time [as the seminal work of Knox (1964) suggests]. But, as Knox (1988) has suggested, we can approach the analysis of disease clusters in two ways. One approach is to define as a cluster any group of cases which is of sufficient size and concentration as to be unlikely to have occurred by chance. This is in essence the approach taken in Openshaw et al's (1987) pioneering work on a geographical analysis machine (GAM). An alternative approach is to argue a priori that the cases are related to each other via a social or biological mechanism (as in a contagious disease) or as "having a common relationship with some other event or circumstance" (Knox, 1988, page 20). Such other events or circumstances might include hypothesised point sources of pollution (for instance, landfill sites or nuclear reprocessing installations) or possible linear sources of environmental impact (for example, busy roads or high-voltage electricity transmission lines). In postulating such environmental associations we would need to set up and evaluate a statistical model to evaluate the hypothesised relationship. As Bithell (1988, page 21) notes, "inferentially, we ought really to be concentrating as far as we can on prior hypotheses". This is what the method we propose allows. We begin by reviewing some alternative approaches to the investigation of disease clusters before setting out this new method. We then explain why we have chosen to model the prevalence of cancer of the larynx and we review what is known about the aetiology of this disease. Results from applying the model to a district in Lancashire are then discussed.

2 Approaches to disease clustering

It is convenient to distinguish between approaches based on counting numbers of cases to be found in each of a set of areal units from those which treat cases as occurring at discrete sites (referenced by a pair of locational coordinates). Our own work falls squarely within the latter type of approach and we simply draw attention to the former, which often involves computing Poisson probabilities for small areas (for instance, see Barnes et al, 1987; Lovett et al, 1990) by using spatial autocorrelation tests to evaluate departures from randomness (Cliff and Haggett, 1988) or by using Bayesian statistics to estimate with use of information about other areas on the map the rates for areal units (Clayton and Kaldor, 1987).

The problem with such area-based approaches, as is well known, is that the results are very much dependent upon the given system of areal units (Openshaw, 1984). The techniques may fail to detect 'real' clusters through which one or more boundaries pass. Further, from the point of view of visualisation we almost always rely on administrative units which are arbitrary in size and shape and are not defined in terms of population at risk. This has led some authors (most recently, Selvin et al, 1988) to construct cartograms in which areal units are deformed such that the represented areas are proportional in size to population. The transformation equalises density and the locations of disease cases may be carried across onto the transformed map. Selvin et al (1988, page 218) give a useful hypothetical example that reveals how natural 'clustering' of cases on an untransformed map arises simply because of variations in population density and how this clustering vanishes when cases are plotted on the cartogram. Investigating real diseases such as cancers, they calculate as a test statistic the average squared distance among cases and evaluate this under the null hypothesis of randomness.

This approach, then, serves as a link between area-based and point-based methods. The latter require very specific locational information, which will not always be available for reasons of confidentiality. However, when these data are available some method is needed to assess whether case 'clustering' is a function of factors other than variations in population density. One way of doing this is to use data on a control population (matched for factors other than the hypothesised 'risk' variable). Cuzick and Edwards (1990) propose an imaginative approach in which a nearest-neighbour graph is constructed on the set of all points (cases and controls together) and where the test statistic is the count of case–case joins. There are close parallels here with a spatial autocorrelation approach.

Openshaw's GAM (Openshaw et al, 1987) is also a point-pattern analysis technique, though it relies on area-based population census data (at an enumeration district level) for computing expected prevalences. Briefly, a count is made of the number of cases within a circle of fixed radius, and if this exceeds the expected number the circle is plotted on a map. This test is performed for many overlapping circles of the same size, with the procedure repeated for circles of varying radius. Visually, a cluster of cases is recognized by a dense pattern of circles, and Openshaw has used the technique to confirm the existence of a concentration of childhood leukaemia around the Sellafield nuclear reprocessing plant and to reveal the existence of another around Gateshead. Openshaw is quite explicit in his philosophy of how to use GAM, namely as an exploratory tool, "relegating the importance of specifying a hypothesis from a locationally specific to a locationally unspecific form. It is noted that lack of knowledge generally precludes more precise formulations of hypotheses in cancer studies" (Openshaw and Craft, 1988, page 35). He recommends GAM as a search tool, leading to more detailed epidemiological studies when we know which areas to target.

3 A new methodology

Our own approach is set more firmly on a foundation of statistical modelling, and we seek to test an explicit hypothesis, namely whether there is an association between a possible point source of pollution and the distribution of a cancer. We also start from the premise that methods based on discrete areal units are always subject to the criticism that the results are specific to that particular set of units. Rather than being constrained by fixed (though essentially arbitrary) areal units such as wards or enumeration districts, we propose an approach based on spatial point processes (Diggle, 1983). [For a full discussion of this method, see Diggle, 1990].

Let us take a spatial distribution of diagnosed cases of some disease represented geographically as a set of points whose grid references are known residential locations. In the absence of any prior information we might suggest an homogeneous Poisson process with constant intensity, λ, as an appropriate null model for these cases. Of course, given known spatial variations in population density this process is not reasonable a priori and we need to consider an inhomogeneous Poisson process in which $\lambda(x)$ varies with location and whose mean is $\int_A \lambda(x) dx$, where x represents location and A is the area of interest. [Note that x is a vector comprising a pair of of locational coordinates (x_1, x_2).] Suppose that the local intensity of cases is expressed as:

$$\lambda(x) = \rho \lambda_0(x) f(x, \theta) , \qquad (1)$$

where ρ represents the overall prevalence of the disease and $\lambda_0(x)$ represents the spatial variation in local intensity under the null

hypothesis. Let f(.) represent the hypothesis of interest here, namely
that $\lambda(x)$ depends upon distance from a postulated point source of
pollution; θ represents a set of parameters to be estimated. Below, we
choose $f(x; 0) = 1$ so that $\theta = 0$ represents the null hypothesis of no
association between local intensity of cases and the postulated source.
That is to say, if there is no association the intensity of cases is the same
as the intensity of controls, scaled by the overall prevalence of cases.

A log-likelihood, $L(\rho, \theta)$, for θ is given by

$$L(\rho, \theta) = n\ln\rho + \sum_{i=1}^{n} \ln f(x_i, \theta) - \rho \int_A \lambda_0(x) f(x, \theta) . \tag{2}$$

Differentiating with respect to ρ, we obtain a maximum-likelihood
estimate for ρ, $\hat{\rho}$:

$$\frac{\partial L}{\partial \rho} = \frac{n}{\rho} - \int_A \lambda_0(x) f(x, \theta) dx = 0 , \tag{3}$$

$$\hat{\rho} = n \frac{1}{\int_A \lambda_0(x) f(x, \theta) dx} . \tag{4}$$

Inserting this expression for $\hat{\rho}$ into equation (2), we get

$$L(\theta) = -n \ln[\int_A \lambda_0(x) f(x, \theta) dx] + \sum_{i=1}^{n} \ln f(x, \theta) . \tag{5}$$

The problem thus becomes one of trying to estimate the background
intensity function $\lambda_0(x)$, as this is unknown. We could make use of
census data but because these are only available for discrete areal units
we prefer a different approach, that is, to use the observed spatial
distribution of another, more common disease, one which matches the
disease of interest in terms of age–sex structure but which, ideally, is
not associated with the hypothesised point source of pollution. Our
choice of the 'control' disease is discussed below, but let us assume for
the present it is given. We need then to convert the control locations
into a continuous intensity function. This is done by smoothing the
point pattern of control locations.

This smoothing of point patterns has been investigated by Diggle
(1985) and Berman and Diggle (1989), who propose, for any location x:

$$\hat{\lambda}_0(x) = \frac{1}{h^2} \sum_{j=1}^{m} w\left(\frac{x - y_j}{h}\right) , \tag{6}$$

where y_j ($j = 1, ..., m$) are the locations of the m controls and w is a
'kernel function' or radially symmetric probability density function, such
as the Gaussian:

$$w(x) = \frac{1}{2\pi} \exp\left(-\frac{1}{2} x' x\right) . \tag{7}$$

The amount of smoothing is determined by h, which is chosen to minimise the mean square error of $\hat{\lambda}_0(x)$. We then have sufficient information to obtain a maximum-likelihood estimate of the parameter(s) θ and to evaluate the null hypothesis (H_0) that $\theta = 0$. In principle we can say that

$$D(\theta) = 2[L(\hat{\theta}) - L(\theta)] \tag{8}$$

is approximately distributed as χ^2, with degrees of freedom equal to the dimensionality of θ (number of parameters to be estimated).

4 Cancer of the larynx

We seek now to test the hypothesis that cancer of the larynx in a district of Lancashire is associated with proximity to a closed-down industrial waste incinerator. We begin by outlining the background to this empirical study before reviewing what is known of the disease aetiology.

Between 1972 and 1980 an industrial waste incinerator operated at a site about 2 km southwest of the small town of Coppull in Lancashire. The incinerator was used for the disposal of a wide range of waste products, both solids and liquids (such as solvents and oils). During its period of operation there were complaints about noxious smells and about respiratory problems. The opening of the plant preceded the setting up of pollution regulations, under the Control of Pollution Act (1974). Since its closure there have been lingering worries about longer-term ill-health effects, and two of us (Gatrell and Lovett) were asked to conduct a preliminary study of the distribution of cancers throughout the area (Chorley and South Ribble District Health Authority) with a view to suggesting whether there was any map evidence of possible clustering in the vicinity of the incinerator. To this end, we were given postcoded data on 6200 cases of cancer diagnosed between 1974 and 1983—patients who were resident in the District at the time of diagnosis. The full unit postcode can be associated with an Ordnance Survey grid reference by using the Central Postcode Directory—a large computer file that lists all 1.5 million unit postcodes in Britain together with corresponding grid references accurate to 100 m (for further details and commentary on the nature of this postcode matching, see Gatrell, 1989).

We found nothing of interest in most of the maps, save for a rather odd distribution of laryngeal cancer (figure 1). There were only 58 cases of this cancer during the 10-year period and the distribution was sparse, with relatively few cases in the more densely populated areas (such as south Preston, Chorley, and Leyland). However, there were 5 cases in the village of Coppull, 4 of which lay within 1 km of the incinerator and another within about 2 km. We regarded this as suspicious, particularly in view of our prior knowledge of the existence of a possible point source of pollution. It therefore seemed worthwhile to attempt to verify by using a statistical model whether or not there was any evidence for local clustering.

What evidence is there, if any, to link cancer of the larynx to proximity to an incinerator? More precisely, are there any known carcinogens which might be released during the combustion of industrial, especially toxic, wastes?

Kleinsasser (1988) has summarised chemical environmental factors that appear to be implicated in laryngeal cancer aetiology. The evidence comes primarily from occupational studies rather than from those affected outside the workplace, and, as Kleinsasser notes, it is difficult to pinpoint individual noxious agents as causes of laryngeal cancer. However, he refers to polycyclic aromatic hydrocarbons (PAHs) as well-known carcinogens and these are by-products of combustion processes (see also Greenberg, 1988). Asbestos fibres are also considered as a causative factor (Stell and McGill, 1975), and poor disposal of any asbestos wastes may release these into the atmosphere. Kleinsasser also reports on exposure to arsenic, formaldehyde, vinyl chloride, sulphuric acid, cadmium, nickel, and chromate dust as risk factors (see also Flanders et al, 1984). Exposure to mustard gas in the field and in the workplace has been identified as a likely cause of some carcinomas. Last, thermal radiation, as experienced by those working in foundries and coke ovens, is said to be a risk factor, that is, warm air containing "all

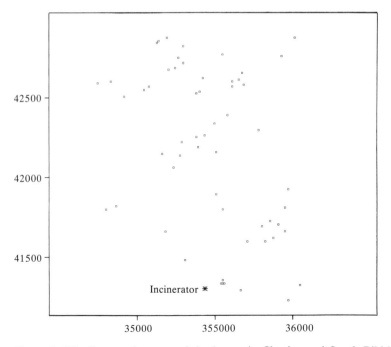

Figure 1. Distributon of cancer of the larynx in Chorley and South Ribble District Health Authority. (Axes refer to the Ordnance Survey grid.)

manner of gases, steam and dust, which may act as carcinogens, although individually they can hardly be identified" (Kleinsasser, 1988, page 18).

Even if we knew the precise details of substances burnt by the incinerator in question during the 1970s and if we had conducted environmental monitoring of stack gases and ground deposition to detect some of the above substances, it would be difficult to infer causal relationships. "The intensity and length of exposure, the age at the time of exposure, and other factors, such as the ubiquitous cigarette smoke, also play a part" (Kleinsasser, 1988, page 18). There is unambiguous evidence that tobacco consumption is the major risk factor in developing the cancer. Burning the tobacco releases tar containing several species of PAHs. Kleinsasser estimates that at least 90% of patients with laryngeal cancer are, or have been, active smokers. Heavy consumption of alcohol is also considered to be a promoting factor in the disease, but one which interacts with smoking to generate an increased risk where both are consumed in excess (Guenel et al, 1988).

All this is to suggest that any attempt to infer causation from a possible point source of pollution is fraught with difficulties. We do not have any information on individuals' smoking behaviour, nor much detail on likely occupational exposure. We do know the age and sex of each case and although the sample (n = 58) is small the age–sex distribution is roughly in line with that for larger samples (figure 2).

The length of time between exposure and diagnosis causes a further difficulty. This time is highly variable, ranging from perhaps 4 or 5 years to 30 years or more (Stell and McGill, 1975, page 516). If it could be demonstrated that the 5 cases close to the incinerator were long-time residents of the areas, with no history of heavy smoking and no evidence of occupational exposure, the argument in favour of the incinerator as a

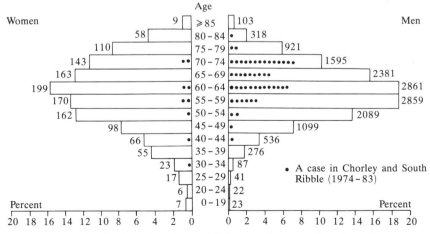

Figure 2. Age distribution of patients with laryngeal cancer (based on European cancer registries). Source: Kleinsasser, 1988.

likely causative factor would be strengthened. We simply do not have enough evidence to argue one way or another.

5 Results

We took data on cancer of the lung (978 observations in our study area) as a variable used to construct the background intensity function, $\lambda_0(\boldsymbol{x})$. We clearly required a variable which is similar to the disease of interest, and in terms of age and sex structure this is the case for these two cancers. Smoking, too, is a major risk factor for both diseases. Alcohol consumption is a risk factor for laryngeal but not for lung cancer, but it is difficult to argue that this introduces a major bias. Strictly speaking, the approach is not valid if lung cancer is associated with the pollution source. If it is, the lung cancer 'controls' are overmatched and the likelihood of finding a significant relationship with proximity to the incinerator is reduced. So we might argue that this particular concern is serious only if the hypothesis of no association is accepted. We reiterate the view that our approach seems preferable to one that uses appropriate age–sex matched controls drawn from areally aggregated census data.

A plot of the lung cancers (figure 3) reveals clumps of local intensity that correspond to centres of population (primarily south Preston, Leyland, and Chorley). We smoothed this point pattern according to the method outlined above, using $h = 0.30$ (figure 4). This is the value which minimises the estimated mean square error of $\lambda_0(\boldsymbol{x})$, as the plot of this error against h reveals (figure 5).

In order for the model to fit [equation (1) above], we needed to specify an explicit functional form for $f(\boldsymbol{x};\ \theta)$. We used:

$$f(d) = 1 + \alpha \exp(-\beta d^2)\,, \tag{9}$$

where d is distance from the incinerator, and α and β are parameters to be estimated. The use of a squared-distance term is arbitrary, but we felt this appropriately reflected a likely pollution-plume effect. The parameter α reflects the risk at source, and β represents variation with distance. Clearly, if there is no distance effect then $f(d) = 1$ and our estimate of the intensity of laryngeal cancer at a point is simply the estimated intensity of lung cancer, scaled by ρ [equation (1)].

The likelihood function [see equation (5)] was evaluated, and maximum-likelihood estimates of α and β were generated. The maximised log-likelihood is -394.593, which is to be compared with a log-likelihood of -399.360 under the null hypothesis. Evaluation of twice the difference between these values as χ^2, distributed with 2 degrees of freedom ($\chi^2_{2,\,0.05} = 5.99$) suggests that H_0 is to be rejected. There are many possible combinations of α and β which generate a maximised log-likelihood close to -394.593 (figure 6), and so it is difficult to be precise about an estimated function $f(d)$. One possibility, where $\hat{\alpha} = 25.26$ and

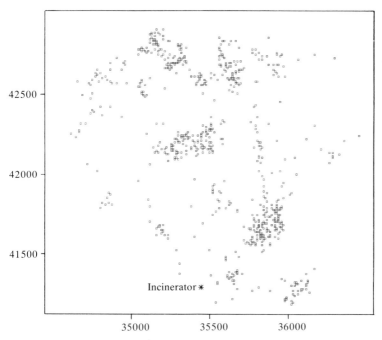

Figure 3. Distribution of cancer of the lung in Chorley and South Ribble District Health Authority. (Axes refer to the Ordnance Survey grid.)

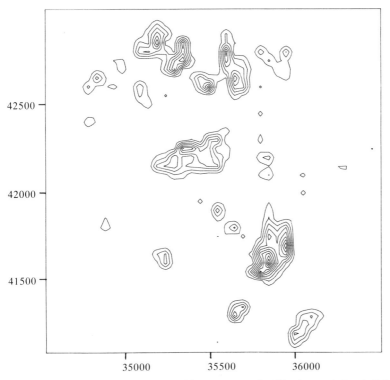

Figure 4. Smoothed distribution of lung cancers in Chorley and South Ribble District Health Authority; $h = 0.3$ km.

$\hat{\beta} = 0.952$, is sketched in figure 7, but as the surface of the log-likelihood would suggest, values of $10 \leqslant \hat{a} \leqslant 200$ and $0.5 \leqslant \hat{\beta} \leqslant 2.5$ are all plausible.

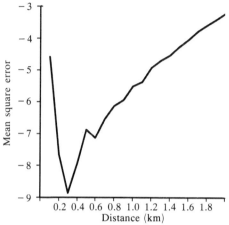

Figure 5. Mean square error, t, of the background intensity function, $\lambda_0(x)$, as a function of distance.

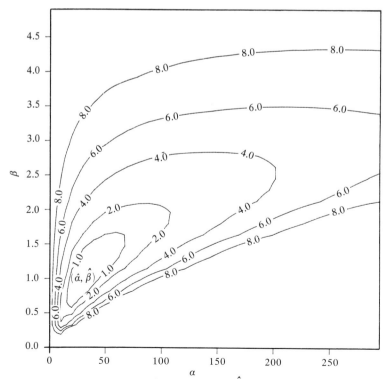

Figure 6. Contour plot of $D(\alpha, \beta) = 2L(\hat{a}, \hat{\beta}) - L(\alpha, \beta)\}$. Values of (α, β) within the 6.0 contour constitute an approximate 95% confidence region.

The reason for this uncertainty is the fact that there is a very marked clump of cases within about 2 km of the incinerator and little else within a radius of 5 km.

We conclude that proximity to the incinerator has some effect on the prevalence of laryngeal cancer. However, we should caution that we are indeed dealing with very small numbers. Taking the 5 cases within 2 km of the incinerator and removing one of these from the analysis, we generate a difference between the maximised and null log-likelihoods, which just fails to reach significance at the 0.05 level [$D(\theta) = 5.82$]. Removing two cases, we reduce $D(\theta)$ to 2.96. The addition of an imaginary case in the same general area gives $D(\theta) = 12.95$. Clearly, then, we cannot escape the fact that we are dealing with small numbers.

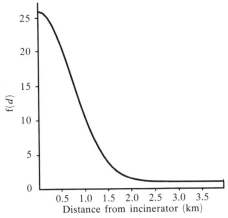

Figure 7. The estimated function of distance, $f(d)$.

6 Conclusions

In geographical epidemiology, there is always a possibility of plotting cases of a disease, detecting 'clusters' by eye, and looking for a possible source of environmental pollution to which one seeks to relate cases. This retrospective formulation of hypotheses is to be studiously avoided. What we have done is to suggest that the distribution of laryngeal cancer may be associated with proximity to an individual waste incinerator. Clearly, we need now to test this hypothesis in other areas. To this end we are extending the study to examine laryngeal and lung cancer in the North West Regional Health Authority as a whole and we will assess other incinerators as possible sources. Obvious candidates here are hospital incinerators—problems with which nationally have already been identified (NSCA, 1988).

We shall also explore the possibility of varying the location of the putative source of pollution within the present study area. This parallels

Openshaw's GAM approach and will generate a surface of maximum-likelihood estimates across the map. It will then be possible to assess the significance of the incinerator relative to other locations on the map. It is also possible in principle to extend the method to incorporate other explanatory variables, where these too are measured at point locations. We see the method we have outlined here in having potentially wide applicability in geographical epidemiology, notably in testing hypotheses concerning the possible impact of nuclear installations on human health.

Acknowledgments. The data come from the North West Regional Cancer Registry, courtesy of Professor A Smith, University of Manchester. We are grateful to Doctor S Sivayoham (Specialist in Community Medicine, Chorley and South Ribble Health Authority) for his support. Doctor A Sudell, Senior Registrar in Community Medicine, Preston Health Authority, has acted as an excellent sounding board throughout this work.

References
Alexander F E, Cartwright R A, McKinney P M, 1988, "A comparison of recent statistical techniques of testing for spatial clustering: preliminary results", in *Methodology of Enquiries into Disease Clustering* Ed. P Elliot (Small Area Health Statistics Unit, London School of Hygiene and Tropical Medicine, 25 Keppel Street, London WC1) pp 23–33
Barnes N, Cartwright R A, O'Brien C, Roberts B, Richards J D G, Hopkinson J M, Chorlton J, Bird C C, 1987, "Variation in lymphoma incidence within Yorkshire Health Region" *British Journal of Cancer* **55** 81–84
Berman M, Diggle P J, 1989, "Estimating weighted integrals of the second-order intensity of a spatial point process" *Journal of the Royal Statistical Society, B* **51** 81–92
Bithell J, 1988, "Discussion of paper by Knox (1988)", in *Methodology of Enquiries into Disease Clustering* Ed. P Elliot (Small Area Health Statistics Unit, London School of Hygiene and Tropical Medicine, 25 Keppel Street, London WC1) page 21
Clayton D, Kaldor J, 1987, "Empirical Bayes estimates for use in disease mapping" *Biometrics* **43** 671–681
Cliff A D, Haggett P, 1988 *Atlas of Disease Distributions: Analytical Approaches to Epidemiological Data* (Basil Blackwell, Oxford)
Control of Pollution Act, 1974 *Public General Acts—Elizabeth II, 1974* chapter 40 (HMSO, London)
Cuzick J, Edwards R, 1990, "Tests for spatial clustering of events for inhomogeneous populations" *Journal of the Royal Statistical Society, B* **52** 73–104
Diggle P J, 1983 *Statistical Analysis of Spatial Point Patterns* (Academic Press, London)
Diggle P J, 1985, "A kernel method for smoothing point process data" *Applied Statistics* **34** 138–147
Diggle P J, 1990, "A point process modelling approach to raised incidence of a rare phenomenon in the vicinity of a pre-specified point" *Journal of the Royal Statistical Society, A* **153** (forthcoming)

Elliot P (Ed.), 1988 *Methodology of Enquiries into Disease Clustering* (Small Area Health Statistics Unit, London School of Hygiene and Tropical Medicine, 25 Keppel Street, London WC1)

Flanders W D, Cann C I, Rothman K H, Fried M P, 1984, "Work-related risk factors for laryngeal cancer" *American Journal of Epidemiology* **119** 23–32

Gatrell A C, 1989, "On the spatial representation and accuracy of address-based data in the United Kingdom" *International Journal of Geographical Information Systems* **3** 335–348

Greenberg A, 1988, "Analyses of polycyclic aromatic hydrocarbons", in *Toxic Air Pollution: A Comprehensive Study of Non-criteria Air Pollutants* Eds P J Lioy, J M Daisey (Lewis, Chelsea, MI) pp 91–121

Guenel P, Chastang J F, Luce D, Leclerc A, Brugere J, 1988, "A study of the interaction of alcohol drinking and tobacco smoking among French cases of laryngeal cancer" *Journal of Epidemiology and Community Health* **42** 350–354

Kleinsasser O, 1988 *Tumours of the Larynx and Hypopharynx* (Thienne Medical Publications, New York)

Knox E G, 1964, "The detection of space–time interactions" *Applied Statistics* **13** 25–29

Knox E G, 1988, "Detection of clusters", in *Methodology of Enquiries into Disease Clustering* Ed. P Elliot (Small Area Health Statistics Unit, London School of Hygiene and Tropical Medicine, 25 Keppel Street, London WC1)

Lovett A A, Gatrell A C, Bound J P, Harvey P W, Whelan A R, 1990, "Congenital malformations in the Fylde Region of Lancashire, England, 1957–73" *Social Science and Medicine* **30** 103–109

NSCA, 1988 *Air Pollution from Crown Property* (National Society for Clean Air, 136 North Street, Brighton BN1 1RG)

Openshaw S, 1984 *CATMOG 38: The Modifiable Areal Unit Problem* (Geo Books, Norwich)

Openshaw S, Charlton M, Wymer C, Craft A W, 1987, "A mark 1 geographical analysis machine for the automated analysis of point data sets" *International Journal of Geographical Information Systems* **1** 335–338

Openshaw S, Craft A, 1988, "Some recent developments of the geographical analysis machine concept", in *Methodology of Enquiries into Disease Clustering* Ed. P Elliot (Small Area Health Statistics Unit, London School of Hygiene and Tropical Medicine, 25 Keppel Street, London WC1) pp 35–40

Selvin S, Merrill D, Schulman J, Sacks S, Bedell L, Wong L, 1988, "Transformations of maps to investigate clusters of disease" *Social Science and Medicine* **26** 215–222

Stell P M, McGill T, 1975, "Exposure to asbestos and laryngeal carcinoma" *Journal of Laryngology* **89** 513–517

Automating the Search for Cancer Clusters: A Review of Problems, Progress, and Opportunities

S OPENSHAW
University of Newcastle upon Tyne

1 Introduction

There are 2 principal ways of tackling the problem of cancer clustering. The first is to use an exploratory data analysis in which a geographically referenced disease data base is searched for evidence of clustering without any a priori hypothesis of where to look or what to look for. This is not an easy task and the statistical methodology used must be able to distinguish between real and spurious patterns and associations. The objective is to generate hypotheses by 'letting the data speak' which would then need to be tested for validity by using different data. The second approach is the more traditional scientific paradigm in which a study is designed to confirm or refute a genuine a priori hypothesis (Davies and Inskip, 1986). It is particularly important in a hypothesis-testing study that the data used to test the hypothesis are independent of the data used to generate it. In addition, various sources of bias need to be eliminated through the use of a predefined analysis structure to avoid the unintentional selection of the analysis domain (namely geographical study region, time period, disease grouping, and age–sex categorisations) through prior knowledge of the data (Wakeford et al, 1989). These 2 different approaches may be characterised by the 2 extremes of my geographical analysis machine (GAM) (Openshaw et al, 1987; 1988a; 1988b) and Kinlen's rural-newcomer hypothesis (Kinlen, 1988; 1989).

In practice it is extremely difficult to specify genuine a priori hypotheses. Kinlen's approach possesses considerable statistical power. From a traditional scientific point of view, it is beyond reproach; yet from the perspective of data analysis it is simultaneously beguiling and potentially deficient. There is no process knowledge to support the hypothesis, the data used are 'old' and probably unreliable, and the categorisation of rural new towns in Kinlen (1989) is not accurate. There is also some prospect that the results might be explained by an alternative hypothesis. Cancer rates are thought to be least reliable in rural areas of rapid population change because the denominator counts from the census provide a poor (owing to lag effects) representation of the population at risk. The elevated rates Kinlen (1989) reports to support his hypothesis may therefore merely reflect this data artifact.

The great difficulty in specifying genuine a priori hypotheses of processes that cause cancer puts great reliance on a more exploratory approach. Furthermore, it is known that cancer causation is highly complex, multifactored, and possessed of a strong stochastic component which makes the task of hypothesis generation extremely hard. It is also unrealistic to expect that medical researchers are going to be able to specify many or even any good sensible a priori hypothesis to be refuted or confirmed in subsequent tests. It would be very nice but it is also probably inpracticable given current medical knowledge. Last, it is still an open question as to whether 'real' cancer clusters actually exist. It is seemingly necessary to try and at least answer this question by making a spatial analysis of whatever data are available as a means of generating clues for further study.

In the era of geographical information systems (GIS) this approach requires an ability to explore systematically and comprehensively whatever geographically referenced medical data bases happen to exist for evidence of patterns and relationships without being hindered either by a lack of prior knowledge about what to expect or by prejudices about the nature of the patterns and relationships thought to exist. It is recognised that the available data will seldom be ideal, that this search task is complicated, and that the preliminary results may well be lacking in power. Additionally, there are real limits to how useful a purely spatial approach can be in an area where virtually all the available variables are either irrelevant or else proxies for other unknown variables. Nevertheless, there is a strong pragmatic requirement for something to be done.

1.1 Key questions

In the United Kingdom, the Black Report (Black, 1984) can be credited with drawing attention to the problem of determining whether certain cancers cluster. The problem can be further rationalised as a search for confident answers to 5 difficult questions:

(1) Is there any strong evidence of cancer clusters?
(2) Where are these possible clusters located?
(3) What is the probability that some or all the clusters are spurious?
(4) What is the probability of a real cluster occuring at a specified location (that is, town or subregion)?
(5) What socioeconomic and/or environmental variables might be associated with the excess incidence of cancer?

There are obviously many different ways of tackling these questions. A variety of geographical and statistical methods could be employed. Indeed this whole problem area is now part of the statistical research agenda (see the special issue of the *Journal of the Royal Statistical Society, Series A* , 1989, volume 152) but so far only a little progress seems to have been made, mainly on questions (1) and (2).

One explanation for the lack of statistical progress in the 5 years since the Black Report is that these questions are exceedingly difficult to answer and it is only recently that spatial statisticians have started to take an interest in this area. Another factor is a realisation that perhaps existing statistical technology is inadequate for the tasks that have been set and that a delay is inevitable as new methods are developed. Another view would be that perhaps it is the deficiencies of data and not methodology that are also a restraining factor. A further consideration is the strong interaction that exists between the geographical and statistical aspects of the problem which makes it difficult for unidisciplinary approaches to succeed. For instance, there is little point in developing a soundly based statistical technique which is strongly dependent on the prior definition of a study region (for example, see Cuzick and Edwards, 1990), or else only concerns itself with large rather than small geographic areas (Clayton and Kaldor, 1987). It is also unreasonable to expect that sensible results can be obtained by applying sophisticated statistical methods to any arbitrary set of geographical areas such as local authority districts (for example, see Cook-Mozaffari et al, 1987) and then putting considerable effort into the detailed interpretation of the results. Other problems concern the need to handle positional uncertainty in the geographic data and the existence of various sources of bias in disease data. None of this makes for either easy analysis or definitive results. It might appear very easy to declare simply that neither the analytic technology nor the available medical data are at present adequate for detailed investigations of cancer clustering. Although there is a degree of truth in such a view, there is also a very strong imperative to abstract as much as possible from whatever data happen to exist, to try and answer genuine public concerns, and to see whether it is possible to provide any spatial clues to disease aetiology. Surely it should be possible with current analytical and computer technology to do something even if the results are likely to remain of a preliminary rather than of a definitive nature.

It is with this objective in mind, that I review some of the recent developments associated with an approach to the problem based on one particular type of geographical analysis. In section 2 I describe the original concept of an automated analysis tool as a descriptive cluster-spotting device. In section 3 I try to put the original prototype procedure in a more general context. In section 4 I look at some of the results that have been achieved, and in section 5 I offer some concluding comments.

2 Developing a mark 1 GAM
2.1 Some basic principles
From a geographical perpsective the GIS revolution is seen as creating the need for new spatial analysis technology to cope with situations in which the data are rich but the theory is poor. This model is seen as being particularly appropriate to spatial epidemiology. The original idea involved creating a relatively hypothesis-free exploratory search technique that can scan (some people say 'trawl') a geographically referenced disease data base in search of evidence of spatial patterning in the form

of clusters. The search takes place in geographic space but could be extended to handle time. This generic procedure was termed a geographical analysis machine (Openshaw et al, 1987). It is suggested that this type of spatial analytical engine should possess the following characteristics.

(a) It must have the ability to make use of the finest level of available geographical information. For example, there is no point in studying ward-scale data when census enumeration district information exists, or of studying enumeration districts when unit postcode data become available. In fact the GIS revolution is increasing dramatically the spatial detail of the available information for spatial epidemiology (see table 1). This means that large values of N can be handled and that the spatial analysis technology is not limited by data size.

(b) The procedure should be boundary free in that it should not be overly dependent on a particular set of arbitrary areal units for its objects of analysis. There is an advantage in using zones which have an equal expectation of disease (COMARE, 1988; Urquhart et al, 1989) but the resulting zonal map patterns used for analysis have to be believable and cannot be based on random geography.

(c) It should be able to handle rather than ignore the special features associated with spatial data. Of particular concern is the presence of positional and representational uncertainty in geographic information and the consequential need to incorporate error handlers explicitly in the analysis procedures rather than to assume that these effects can be ignored.

(d) The search process should be locationally systematic and comprehensive to ensure that all areas are examined and that all locations are treated equally. This avoids the problem of post hoc model construction resulting from prior knowledge of the data, as such knowledge is rendered irrelevant owing to the comprehensive and automated nature of the search.

(e) Automation is needed to cope with characteristics (a) and (d). It also offers some insurance against user interference in the analysis.

Table 1. Numbers and types of geographic data available for Northern England.

Type of areal unit	Number of units	Type of geograhic reference
Counties	8	boundary information
Disticts	54	boundary information
Census wards	1272	boundary information
Census enumeration districts[a]	16237	100 m point references
Unit postcodes[a]	178500	10 m point references
Households[a]	2855248	1 m point references

[a] The geographical analysis machine can work at this scale.

Automation is possible because of the rapidly increasing power of computer hardware which opens up the prospect of a new style of spatial analysis.

(f) The results should be communicable to the user. Cancer, especially in children, is a highly emotive subject, and the analyses need to be capable of being easily understood. The map offers a very useful communication device. The counterview that statistical encryption is in fact a very desirable means of suppressing information in areas that may cause public alarm is not tenable.

(g) There should be some means of assessing the significance or likely importance of the results. An interpretative mechanism is needed for providing the end user with advice as to the meaningfulness of any clusters that are identified. In particular, are they a matter of interest or a cause for possible concern? This requirement also reflects the need to distinguish between potentially real and spurious results and requires that some means must exist to 'clean up' the map patterns to leave a clear message.

(h) The behaviour of the method should be known under synthetic conditions. Ideally, some assessment needs to be made of its statistical power in order to reduce the risks of imparting meaning to random variation.

(i) Finally, there should be some advice about how to utilise the technology. For instance, there is a major difference beween a purely descriptive exercise which aims at identifying possible areas of interest as map description and the more rigorous testing of statistical hypotheses which requires a precise measure of statistical significance.

Automated search methods need to be 'robust' to the various sources of uncertainty that tend to characterise disease data and yet still be sensitive enough to detect localised deviation from what may otherwise be a spatially random pattern. It is noted that there is little benefit in only being able to determine whether or not clustering is present, without any mechanism for identifying where it is located. Whether it is possible to meet these objectives is a matter for debate. However, if such a system can be developed then there is little doubt that it could well be of immense value both for the retrospective analysis of historic patterns of disease and, more usefully, as the basis for a real-time disease monitoring system. The challenge is set and the task is how best to meet it.

There are clearly a number of different approaches to this objective. The interest in searching for clusters is a logical extension of the mapping of a disease. It is important to know 'where to look' as knowledge of the spatial distribution of disease can sometimes provide clues about what may be causing the local excess and thus act as a focus for a more detailed subsequent investigation; however, spatial analysis can never prove causation, it can only identify potentially interesting and unusual empirical regularities. To some extent, it is possible to view Clayton and Kaldor (1987) as seeking to approach this objective from a mapping perspective by using empirical Bayes statistics to handle problems of data unreliability and by incorporating spatial autocorrelation as a means of reducing the dependency of the results on the choice of a particular arbitrary set of areal units. The original GAM adopted a different approach to essentially the same objective and may well offer a complementary geographic procedure.

2.2 A prototype GAM

The above list of design principles [characteristics (a) to (i)] was enumerated subsequent to rather than prior to the development of a prototype GAM (see Openshaw et al, 1987; 1988a; 1988b). That first attempt at building an automated cluster-spotting machine as a surveillance tool was a geographer's response to the practical problems of searching a cancer data base for evidence of spatial clustering under circumstances where an exploratory approach was obligatory owing to the absence of sensible or properly specified a priori hypotheses. It was a reflection of an underlying belief that there were many new opportunities there for the development and application of a more heavily geographically biased and computer automated style of spatial analysis than was traditionally popular in geography and regional science.

The basic idea that resulted in the development of the first GAM was very simple and was a direct result of reading Wilkie's evidence at the 1986–87 public inquiry into the Dounreay Fast Reactor Reprocessing Plant (Wilkie, 1986). There the complaint was made that the evidence presented at that inquiry by the Information Services Division of the Scottish Health Service Common Services Agency was biased by an unfortunate, albeit unintentional, combination of boundary gerrymandering and post hoc testing of hypotheses. It is noted that, in that study, population and cancer data were obtained for a circular study region and a Poisson probability was used to assess whether the observed number of cancers could have occurred by chance. With this technique there are a number of key operational decisions which may have a major impact on the results: (1) the selection of a point source to be investigated on the basis of a prior hypothesis; (2) the prior selection of a particular radius for the circular study region for which a measure of significance is to be obtained; (3) the prior selection of a specific time period for the study; and (4) the prior selection of either a particular disease or grouping of diseases.

These problems are quite common and in various forms have often characterised studies of cancer clustering. In essence there is no obvious solution other than to resort to massively subjective prior specifications of all the key analysis-domain parameters. The problems reflect the deficiencies of scientific method and statistical technology. The preferred solution is to automate the entire process and then to explore systematically the universe of results that can be obtained by identifying and examining all combinations of the various operational decisions and then try to live with the consequences. Instead of examining only 1 or 2 locations thought to be of particular a priori interest, why not examine all locations? Instead of specifying a specific radius, why not examine a wide spectrum of alternative radii? Instead of selecting a particular time subgrouping why not examine all alternatives, and do likewise for the various disease categorisations considered relevant? With modern computers this type of brute-force approach is feasible and there is no longer any need to be restricted to a manual style of analysis; the back-of-envelope and hand-calculator era of exploratory data analysis has no place here.

However, there are a number of problems in adopting this style of analysis. Particular mention is made of: (1) the need to evaluate perhaps several millions of test statistics for circles, (2) the need to take into account the locational and representational uncertainties implicit in the geographic data being analysed, (3) the complexity of multiple nonindependent significance testing, (4) the dependency of the results on the (unknown) power of whatever test statistic is used as a pattern detector by the search engine, and (5) its sensitivity to the geometry of the spatial search window. Because it avoided some of these extremely difficult-to-answer questions the original GAM was considered to be a geodescriptive tool rather than a statistical technique. The formal hypothesis testing of classical statistics was reduced to a descriptive filter, with the emphasis focused on the descriptive and suggestive nature of the results. Indeed, the use of the GAM as a map descriptive tool is entirely reasonable and may in fact be a good place to stop!

The first of the 5 problems can be overcome either by extended run times or by coding the procedure for a supercomputer. The second problem is handled by a form of autosensitivity analysis with overlapping circles. The other problems were initially ignored because the original limited objective was to develop what was considered to be a purely geographical pattern descriptive technique which put less emphasis on these latter aspects than a more statistical approach would have required. It was also thought that they could be explored via simulation at a later date. The aim was merely to identify potentially anomalous locations to be investigated further with use of a different style of analysis.

The basic idea of taking a particular generic hypothesis [namely, the probability that the observed number of cancers within a circle of radius r at point (x, y) could have occurred by chance] and then of building an analysis engine by generalising the spatial and locational components can be made operational in a number of ways. In the route selected for the initial GAM there are 4 key components: (1) a means of generating the universe of hypotheses of a particular generic type; (2) a means of detecting patterns which involves a test statistic and a significance assesment procedure; (3) a means of visualising the results as a map;

and (4) a GIS to handle all the requests for retrieval of spatial data. I have, with others, provided a full description of these aspects in another paper (Openshaw et al, 1987) and so I repeat only scant details here.

The one key operational decision that needs to be made concerns the nature of the generic hypothesis, although 'hypothesis' is probably not the right term for something which is essentially being used as a screening device. In the GAM a circular region of interest (reflecting its historic origins) is used and the concern is with identifying the subset of all circles that have a sufficient excess of cancer counts to be viewed as different from what would have been expected had the cancer of interest been distributed in a spatially random manner throughout the population at risk in the study region. This assessment is made by using an analytical Poisson calculation. For the range of values encountered here there is no need to use Fisher's exact test.

The locational component of the generic hypothesis is varied in a systematic manner by covering the study region with a lattice. Circles of a given radius are generated about each lattice intersection. The lattice is spaced sufficiently closely relative to the radius of the circles being examined, so that the circles overlap by a large degree. Experiments suggest that a lattice spacing of 0.2 circle radii is suitable, but any small value could be used. It is important that these pseudocircles overlap in order to provide a good discrete approximation to a consideration of all point locations within a particular study region and to allow for edge effects in the geographic data retrieval for circular regions, caused by a mixture of representational and positional uncertainty in the 2-dimensional point references used to represent the data. The inclusion and exclusion of data points near the boundary of a circle may cause spurious patterns to appear. Additionally, because both the population at risk and the cancer data are related to 2-dimensional spatial objects which are represented by centroidal point references, the circles are not really circles but are represented by the irregular boundary of the containing spatial objects. It is important, therefore, that the same spatial representation is used for both sets of data. Finally, the circles need to overlap in order to offer a form of autosensitivity analysis of these edge effects. This is a very important point that affects the use of spatial statistics on this type of data. It is currently unknown what effects locational fuzziness has on many statistical methods, yet it is an endemic characteristic of this type of spatial data. However, because the circles overlap, the resulting significance assessment for neighbouring circles is not necessarily independent. This defect is thought likely to make the GAM a very sensitive pattern detector, which may or may not be a desirable property, depending on its propensity to produce false positives. On the other hand, it does at least attempt to incorporate uncertainty in geographic data and at the time the GAM was being developed this was considered to be just as important.

The scale component of the generic hypothesis is easily handled. Having exhaustively evaluated all circles of a given radius, we can merely increase the radius a little, change the lattice spacing and thus the circle centroids, and then restart the analysis. This procedure is then repeated for a range of circle sizes; typically from 1 km to 30 km radii in increments of 1 km. The lower limit of 1 km reflects the resolution of the data (namely, point references are accurate to 100 m). This should be specified prior to any analysis.

The final components in the GAM are the GIS and the map display system. The former is necessary to allow point data to be retrieved efficiently for each of the million or so circles of varying sizes. In the GAM, originally a recursive-tree-based multipath, multidimensional data structure was used, and was known as a K-D-B tree. This allowed the data to be stored on disk and thus permitted migration into a microenvironment at a later date. It also allowed fast and efficient spatial data retrievals for circular search regions.

The reliance on the map as the final output from the GAM and as a visual representation of pattern may appear a little strange to nongeographers. However, it is quite acceptable to use a map-based evaluation of results as the GAM was originally considered to be a descriptive technique. The original GAM merely showed maps based on all circles judged to be individually significant at some small statistical threshold. The circles shown on the maps had individual Poisson probabilities of less than 0.002, but it is important to note that this was not the correct significance of the whole flock of circles occuring by chance. It was conjectured that if the clustering of circles was sufficiently intense then it would be unlikely to be random, although at the time no measure of overall significance could be attached to it. This did not seem to matter because the objective was to determine where to focus subsequent, more detailed investigations. Indeed, for the results to be deemed of 'medical significance' there would have to be other corroborative evidence. So the risk of statistical type 1 errors was to be reduced by a combination of informed commonsense and prior knowledge based on other evidence and was not reliant solely on the power of the significance test used in the GAM. This informal extrastatistical validation process is obviously important but often overlooked.

However, because the circles overlapped there were problems of double counting; some circles referred to the same data. Reliance on an eyeball interpretation of map patterns may appear unscientific and arbitrary, but maps are very useful devices for communicating results and as a basis for further speculation about what patterns may or may not be present. It was conjectured that any dense, localised concentration of circles that survive the hurdle of significance assessment will provide a useful visual indication of spatial clustering. The ability to identify all areas within the study region where a null hypothesis appears to be breaking down is considered to be a very useful feature. It is also useful to be able to determine the full geographic extent of these patterns rather than to restrict the analysis only to areas near observed cancer cases or around a priori identified putative sources of pollution. The task of assessing the overall significance of the map pattern of circles was thought to be best left to subsequent analysis by different methods. To this extent, the GAM can be regarded as a hypothesis generator and a descriptive mapping technique. This restricted objective of identifying areas where further research might be worthwhile is quite reasonable and is all that might be expected from a spatial analysis technique.

As is now well known, the early GAM application to leukaemia data for Northern and North West England showed the expected Seascale cluster but with a surprising and seemingly even larger Gateshead–Tyneside cluster. The dense concentrations of overlapping circles that were produced were compared with other qualitatively far-less-dense patterns of circles which are thought to be of no great interest. For instance, it is possible to identify various edge effects and other seemingly spurious results. Comparisons with other cancers not thought to cluster tended to support this intuitive interpretation. However, there is no means of knowing what is and what is not an interestingly dense concentration of significant circles, and the end result of this original GAM was basically a map that was difficult to interpret. Were the flocks of overlapping circles a matter of research interest or a matter of public concern? The purpose in presenting these GAM cluster maps was primarily descriptive. The GAM certainly offered a relatively unbiased view of those parts of the study region where there appeared to be some evidence of spatial clustering, as witnessed by the presence of a large number of circles. The maps provided a framework that was informative and suggested possibilities for further investigations. However, whether the patterns they contained were 'real' and not chance occurrences can be determined only by further validation or by development of a statistical GAM.

2.3 Some reactions to a prototype mark 1 GAM

The first GAM grew out of the GIS revolution and is seemingly the first instance of a spatial analysis method that incorporates a GIS within itself. However, it was clearly labelled as a 'prototype' (see Openshaw et al, 1987). It was intended to demonstrate the feasibility of a new way of searching for cancer clusters in the hope that statisticians might then be able to improve the technology and take it further than perhaps a computational geographer might be able to (Openshaw and Craft, 1989). Sadly, the GAM method generated what might be termed a strong ideological response by some academic statisticians who initially appeared to misunderstand what we were trying to do with the GAM, and they failed to appreciate both the limited nature of the available geographical information and the need for exploratory analysis. Maybe also it was a reaction to the 'not-invented-here' technology and to the labelling of an area of spatial statistics as 'geographical'. So on reflection it is hardly surprising that the original GAM aroused both interest and a degree of controversy, the latter mainly behind the scenes.

The critical response also seemed to reflect the origins of the GAM within geography, the adoption of an extensive computational approach, the claims that were made regarding its powers, and the unsought media attention that the preliminary results attracted. Some statisticians do not like 'machines', and the notion that their statistical analysis skills can somehow be automated by using computers is sometimes difficult to accept. Some of the criticism is undoubtedly justified but some of the reaction was seemingly also a reflection of various less understandable ill-feelings that appear to exist between some geographers and certain statisticians in developing spatial analysis methods. These problems are probably largely avoidable by replacing the word 'statistical analysis' by 'geographical analysis'. The GAM was never perceived to be part of that debate but merely an attempt to answer pressing questions concerning the spatial epidemiology of children with cancer; questions that still seem unanswerable by any other means.

2.4 Some criticisms of the original GAM
No technique is without limitations, and the GAM is no exception. The emphasis placed on those problems thought to exist tends to reflect the statistical and to some extent philosophical standpoint of the inquirer. A list of problems would include: (1) multiple significance testing and, more seriously, the large numbers of circles being examined will inevitably result in a test of low power; (2) the overlapping circles may result in too great a sensitivity to certain types of random pattern; (3) there is no obvious quantitative way of comparing the map patterns formed by clusters of overlapping circles; (4) the power of its pattern detection abilities might well be affected by variations in population density and thus by differences between urban and rural areas; (5) there is no satisfactory statistical basis for the GAM because it is an ad hoc technique; (6) it was perceived to be computationally wasteful; and (7) it exhausts the data thereby preventing subsequent testing of any other hypotheses that might be generated. Besag and Newell (1990) provide a further discussion of some of these aspects.

Problems are not unexpected given the novel nature of the method and the objectives underlying the design. Indeed, it is perhaps too easy to lose faith and dismiss the entire approach as being seductively attractive but fundamentally flawed, and then to return to using more conventional methods which may be similarly, or more, flawed but more comfortable because of their wider acceptance. However, there is no reason why these criticisms cannot be answered by developing GAM variants with different properties. There is a danger of being overcautious and too negative in dealing with new technology and by so doing denying for no good reason access to potentially useful methods of analysis. [For example, see Urquhart et al's (1989) attempt to discredit the method by analogy; other critics operated in a far more vicious nonpublic manner.] Clearly, it is difficult to publish any work in a field where the public-policy significance of the results interacts strongly with basic but as yet unanswered methodological concerns. The point at which you can go public with a new set of results is difficult to determine and any publication in such a sensitive area carries some risk. The use of the words 'prototype' and 'mark 1' in the literature to describe the original GAM reflected these feelings and concerns but at the same time there was sufficient confidence in the preliminary results for them to be published. It would have been a very difficult decision to keep quiet about the Tyneside leukaemia cluster once it had been found and its existence seemed to be supported by other independent corroborative evidence (NRHA, 1989). Indeed, a subsequent research project using entirely different methods identified essentially the same results as the original GAM (see Besag and Newell, 1990). Comparative studies based on Yorkshire data also appear to suggest that the GAM is a fairly sensible method (Alexander et al, 1989). Clearly, the GAM does work even if its statistical properties remain something of a mystery.

3 Generalising the GAM concept

3.1 The emergence of GAM/1+

One urgent task was to speed up the original GAM execution times to allow more experimentation with the technology. The code was tuned for the Cray X-MP/48 supercomputer at the Rutherford Appleton Laboratories. Computer times were further reduced by replacing the repeated computation of Poisson probabilities by a table of critical values. Another requirement was that the GAM should be able to handle the problem of multiple significance testing by use of simulation methods. A Monte Carlo significance-testing procedure was used to provide a precise test of the null hypothesis that the observed number of circles is the same as might be produced by a spatially random distribution of disease. This is equivalent to running the original GAM on 499 (or more) randomly generated sets of cancer data. This required that the original recursive data structure of the K-D-B tree be replaced by something capable of efficient execution on a vector processor. The new data structure had to be both 'vectorisable' and able to handle potentially large numbers of randomly generated distributions of disease. It was obviously better to run the GAM once only and retrieve for each circle 500 cancer counts than it would be to run the GAM 500 times. The fast retrieval of point data for a circular search region is solved by using a hash lookup mapped on to a 2-dimensional bucket data structure. The data are stored in a series of '1 km' data blocks, each of which can be accessed by a hash method. The hash points to the start and end addresses of a set of '100 m', '10 m', or '1 m' data records located in the target 1 km square. These data records are held in memory for fast access and a variable word-size sparse-matrix representation is developed to store the M sets of randomly generated distributions of disease. So effective is this method that very little memory is needed and run times are only 2 or 3 times greater than single GAM run would be. Typical CPU times amount to about 7 minutes on a Cray X-MP/48. These statistical and computational developments made it possible to develop the original GAM further and to run it in a highly economical fashion either within a supercomputer environment or on a multiple processing system or even on a fast workstation.

3.2 The emergence of other GAM variants

The development of a supercomputer version of the GAM and a mechanism for handling the problem of multiple significance testing made it possible to investigate by empirical means the performance and sensitivity of the GAM when it runs on synthetic data of known structure. It also allowed GAM/1+ to be used as a system shell that could be configured in various ways. The basic GAM concept has been extended, therefore, to produce other GAM variants by changing both the nature of the search process and the statistical test criteria.

In GAM/2, the problems caused by using overlapping circles are avoided by switching to a grid lattice. This also allows the use of an analytical correction to handle the problem of multiple significance testing without the need for simulation (Wakeford et al, 1989). This has been operationalised and run on a Cray 2 (see Openshaw et al, 1989). A single run takes about 4 minutes. However, the nonindependence problem returns when multiple lattice sizes are considered and if shifts and/or rotations of the lattice origin are used to represent uncertainty in the data. In the second two cases the system of overlapping circles is replaced merely by a system of overlapping grid-squares.

Obviously various other GAMs can be developed. The GAM/1+ principle has been modified to use circles which have floating radii. In GAM/3 a Bithel and Stone, Poisson maximum statistic is used (Stone, 1988). This has the advantage of being adaptive. The optimal distance is automatically identified and a precise test of significance employed. In GAM/4 the circles around each point are constructed to contain a specific target population rather than to represent a fixed metric distance. The critical values can be determined by using a binomial distribution, although for the range of data values relevant here a Poisson approximation is good enough and easier to handle when covariates are introduced. This approach was inspired by Urquhart's work with zones of approximately equal populations (see COMARE, 1988; Urquhart et al, 1989) and is an attempt to overcome rural–urban differences in population density by ensuring that each circle is comparable in terms of the size of population at risk. In GAM/5 the circle radii are varied to ensure that each contains a target number of cancers. The critical populations can be assessed by using a negative binomial distribution, although in practice a Poisson approximation is again good enough. This method is based on the simplified GAM procedure described by Besag and Newell (1990) but is embedded within a GAM shell. In GAM form it is particularly attractive in that there is clearly a much smaller range of potential cancer count targets than there are target populations. The population and cancer targets would be varied over a range of values to allow scale and size effects to manifest themselves. In all cases simulation is used to handle the problem of multiple significance testing. One problem though is the tendency of this nearest-neighbour method to miss small cancer clusters; for example, Seascale.

A key design decision concerns whether it is necessary to examine a fine grid mesh of locations rather than to concentrate on the observed cancer cases, as recommended by Besag and Newell (1990), in order to reduce computational effort and the problems of multiple testing. The view here is that there is no need to be restrictive. There are occasions when it is important that there is a geographically comprehensive search of a fine mesh of locations within the region of interest, irrespective of where the observed cases are located. This could be over the entire region of interest or restricted to certain regions; for example, a corridor based around a linear feature or near observed cases. If the search process is based on the observed cases only, then the results may underestimate the real extent of the clusters. The problem is also that no one really knows where to look and the search decision needs to be flexible rather than overly restrictive. A further criticism of a pure case-only-based search strategy concerns the need to handle locational error and representational uncertainties inherent in the point referencing of areal objects. Effects of data uncertainty can be handled by 'wobbling' the point data to reflect positional uncertainty, and once this is performed by simulation, then a case-only-based method increasingly converges on a systematic GAM-like search.

3.3 New GAM developments

It would not be difficult to add other GAM/n variants to this list; for instance, the circles could become sectors with a directional component, and there are other test statistics that can be employed; for example, Knox's method (Knox, 1964). There are also variants on search strategy (for instance, grid searches, site-specific searches, random sampling, case-based searches, and searches restricted to various map features such as road buffers or geology). It is useful, therefore, to try and put the emerging GAM/n variants into some overall framework to allow an overview. One way is to classify the various GAM variants in terms of the characteristics of spatial search and the geometry of the search (see table 2). Much of table 2 is empty, to indicate that other GAM variants are possible but have not been developed. Additionally, some other seemingly different methods can be placed within the GAM framework once data uncertainty is taken into account. Indeed, virtually any test statistic might be utilised within the search areas being used by a GAM [for instance, Cuzick and Edwards's (1990) method]. The circles are being used merely as windows for detecting patterns. Likewise a variety of different areal configurations could also be used (for instance, instead of circles, one could use squares, segments of circles, triangles, and rotated rectangles). Finally, a more novel suggestion is to define a set of search areas based on overlaying polygons which represent covariates [for example, irregular areas resulting from the overlay of geology with road buffers and proximity to power cables (see Openshaw et al, 1990].

In all cases so far, the critical test statistic is a count of the total number of significant results (that is, circles or squares) that appear anywhere on the map. This made sense in terms of the logic of the underlying GAM concept. It is also possible to develop a number of alternative measures (see table 3). However, they all share some undesirable properties. In particular, the results reflect whole map patterns (as the statistics are accumulated over the whole study region) and thus reflect directly the definition and size of the study region. This can produce all manner of modifiable study region effects . For instance, an excess of circles in a study restricted to Tyne and Wear may be lost when the whole Northern Region is analysed. These problems can be circumnavigated by purely arbitrary means (for instance, to claim a priori that Tyne and Wear is of interest for some preanalysis reason); however, this is a fairly 'feeble' way of handling a major difficulty in spatial analysis. It might be far better to conclude that 'whole-map' type-1 error probabilities are basically meaningless in spatial analysis because of this dependency on study region and then try to develop procedures that can look within whole map patterns for evidence of more

Table 2. Typology of variants of the geographical analysis machine (GAM).

Pattern of search	Characteristics of search areas			
	distance	Kth nearest neighbour	uniform expectation	adaptive distance
Overlapping circles	GAM/1	GAM/5	GAM/4	GAM/3
Regular grid	GAM/2	–	–	–
Case based	–	–	–	–
Children based	–	–	–	–
Sample points	–	–	–	–
A priori selection	–	–	–	–

localised clustering whilst being invariant with the location of the study region boundary.

One solution is to change the basis of the test by introducing an element of locational specificity. This reflects the view that it is not sufficient to demonstrate that there is an excess of significant results in a study region when the real question is far more focused geographically. Regardless of the outcome for a whole region test, the user may well be amazed to discover that there is a seemingly obvious visual excess of circles in one particular area. The question once again reduces to "What level of significance may be attached to that result?" Strictly speaking, if the question involves a sequential test, then it cannot be answered by the same data that generated the hypothesis. One route is therefore to specify in advance locations where on a priori grounds excesses of circles might have been expected; this then becomes an exercise of testing site-specific hypotheses. A more relevant approach for the GAM in an exploratory context is to estimate the significance that a given extreme observed result for any circle or square might have if it occurred purely by chance, by counting the number of times more extreme results can occur anywhere on the map for a large number of spatially random data distributions given a fixed set of circles or squares. Another alternative is to ask the same question for each observed circle [for example, to count the number of times that spatially random data circles overlap or occur in the vicinity of each observed data circle (or square) and possess a more extreme test statistic]. Provided the test statistic is data independent and the procedure is applied in a uniform manner then there is no reason why a Monte Carlo significance test cannot be used

Table 3. Whole-map pattern statistics.

Statistic
Number of blobs
Number of circles after deduplication
Number of cancers in circles
Number of at-risk population in circles
Ink per cancer
Ink per at-risk population
Total ink used
Mean circle cancer rate in a blob
Mean circles per blob
Mean cancers per blob
Mean at-risk population per blob
Mean cancers per blob circle
Mean at-risk population per blob
Mean at-risk population per blob circle
Mean cancer rate per blob circle
Smallest Poisson probability within blob

here also. One advantage would be a greatly reduced sensitivity to the size of the study region, as the definition of vicinity is independent of the study region boundary.

Furthermore, it might be thought that locationally dependent significance tests become more meaningful and less prone to second-order multiple-testing problems if the objects being examined are changed from circles or squares to something which has perhaps greater natural meaningfuless as a spatial map pattern entity. One suggestion is that the concept of a 'blob' or supercluster provides one such entity. A blob is defined as a collection of spatially overlapping circles or squares. The idea is to reduce a map pattern consisting of K circles to a set of k blobs, where each blob consists of one or more physically overlapping circles. The number of blobs is typically fairly small. The map patterns can be further 'cleaned up' by deleting from each blob all circles that contain duplicate information (that is, based on the same child population and cancers as another circle with a larger radius in the same blob). This 'blob approach' offers another advantage in that the significance test thresholds used to identify mappable circles can be increased to a more typical value (for instance, 0.05 instead of 0.002) without swamping the map with circles. This is thought to be necessary in order to avoid missing clusters and to avoid picking up spurious results. It is also thought that the notion of blobs offers a better representation of the map patterns. They can be applied to noncircular spatial objects and can be employed in a vicinity framework; for instance, define a as the minimum area rectangle that contains a blob and then count the number of times blobs occur there in spatially random data which are more extreme in terms of some blob-based test statistic. A number of test statistics which are descriptive of blob characteristics are shown in table 4.

Another consideration concerns the nature of the statistical testing procedure being used. Basically there are 3 options: no significance test other than as a mapping threshold, as in GAM/1; the use of a Monte Carlo method as a precise test of a specific hypothesis (typically based on 99, 499, or 999 simulations, as used to handle multiple testing in GAM/1 +);

Table 4. Blob statistics.

Statistic
Number of circles after deduplication
Total number of cancers
Total excess of at-risk population
Total at-risk population
Total ink used
Cancer rate
Smallest Poisson probability for any blob circle
Largest excess of at-risk population

and a Monte Carlo estimate of a significance level (based on typically 9999 simulations) attributable to a particular test statistic, as used in GAM/2. The first option is basically what the original GAM offered; that is, all circles that passed an arbitrary, individual probability threshold are mapped. The significance or otherwise of the resulting whole-map pattern is unspecified and reliance is placed on the human eye to identify the spatial patterns and on other evidence to corroborate the results. This is fine as a description of the data provided if it is recognised that the validity of the results must depend on subsequent study at a different scale. The second option merely deals with the problem of multiple significance testing and provides a better guide to the potential meaningfulness of the results by providing a mechanism for estimating type 1 error probabilities for the whole map.

The third option involves considerably greater effort and is an attempt to quantify precisely the significance of a particular result. In a previous paper (Openshaw et al, 1989) it is argued that the best way to achieve this goal is to identify the most extreme result produced for any given set of circles or squares (based on a fixed range of sizes of objects) and then to count the number of times in 9999 simulations of a spatially random disease process that a more extreme result occurs. A study in which this method was used ran for 75 hours of CPU time on a Cray 2. The procedure can be repeated for the second, third, etc most extreme observed result. This is another whole-map pattern statistic which is dependent on the study region boundary, with dilution effects being seen as the area of interest increases. The larger the study region, the more hypotheses to be tested in a comprehensive search and the lower the statistical power of the technique. With this method only the most extreme observed results will probably be capable of detection above a background of random noise. This may well be quite reasonable given the nature of an exploratory search technique and it may be contrasted to the more descriptive geographical approach offered by the original GAM. This problem cannot be avoided but, perhaps, its severity can be reduced by switching the object of analysis from counts of total circles or squares to blobs in the context of what was termed earlier a vicinity analysis. Maybe also there is something to be said in favour of a more artistic and less statistically pure focus in spatial analysis contexts which only aim to provide a guide to further research.

3.4 A GAM(g, m, s) family
This discussion of different analysis options inevitably leads us to the need to try and unify an otherwise very confused picture. The original concept in developing a GAM was to try and provide a generic tool able to handle any and all problems of point data analysis; cancer data were merely the initial area of application. It is interesting, therefore, to try and integrate all the GAMs into a single framework. In the previous

discussion about GAM developments, 3 key characteristics were recognised, with a few options under each. These key decisions involve the choice of: (1) spatial search configuration, (2) map significance assessment, and (3) search strategy. The alternatives under each are listed in table 5.

In the style of Box–Jenkins, it is, then, possible to parameterise the GAM with a parameter for each of these key choices; thus g represents the geometry of the search objects used to search for clusters; m stands for the significance assessment options; and s represents the search strategy. The other options regarding the choice of test statistic and the use of measures of blob or vicinity map pattern are either self-evident or else common to all modes of use. For example, the extension to handle space–time events is equivalent to using a cylinder rather than a circular search geometry. With this GAM family notation, Besag and Newell's method becomes a GAM $(3, 1, 3)$, Stone's method becomes a GAM $(2, 2, 2)$, Urquhart's method is a GAM$(4, 2, 2)$, and the original GAM is a GAM$(1, 1, 1)$. Obviously the list can be extended and many of the methods can be represented by a single generic program. This is useful because it emphasises the overall similarity of the various GAM-like methods and provides a framework for further experimentation.

Table 5. Key search parameters in the geographical analysis machine.

Parameter

Search configuration, g:
    geometric (circles, squares, triangles, and so on)
    multiple geometrics
    cancer count
    approximate equality of population
    polygon overlay

Assessment of map significance, m:
    none
    hypothesis testing
    significance assessment

Search strategy, s:
    locationally comprehensive
    a priori site specific
    case based

---

4 Some experiments with a GAM(1, 1, 1) method

4.1 Generation of synthetic data

The various members of the GAM(g, m, s) family can now be applied to real leukaemia data and the results examined. However, there still remains a lack of knowledge about the statistical power of the technology and the need to perfect the concept of using blobs and vicinity analysis.

This can be done by experimentation but not with 'real' data because the 'true' result is unknown and there is no real basis for choosing between the alternatives. It seems advisable, therefore, to test out the new methods on synthetic data where the structure of the data is known. One problem with such an approach is knowing what assumptions to make regarding the type of spatial pattern likely to be representative of leukaemia. A number of different models might be assumed; for instance, point based, a contagious process, and a general model of increased area incidence.

In this paper only a simple point model is considered. It is assumed that there is a point around which cancer incidence is some function of distance. A total of 3 distance bands are used: 0 km to 2.5 km, 2.5 km to 5 km, and 5 km to 10 km, with incidence rates which are, respectively, 16, 8, and 4 times greater than expected. The distribution of cases within these areas is still random amongst the population at risk but has a mean incidence related to distance from the point source. A final subjective parameter is the number of cases of cancer to be treated as being associated with a point source. The simplest assumption here was to partition the total number of cancers into 2 parts; spatially random according to a global incidence rate, and associated with one source (or more). The percentage assumed to be point-cluster related was varied, and included 25%, 10%, 5%, 2.5%, 2%, and 1% of total cases. In this study, 2 point-locations are considered; a rural site (Sellafield) and an urban site (Gateshead). Ideally, a large number of random simulations should be performed around each location and the results examined to yield power curves. Here the results of a preliminary study are reported which involve only one simulation for each assumption. Further simulations have been performed and support these findings.

4.2 Results from the synthetic data

The GAM(1, 1, 1) method is applied, with 499 spatially random data sets being used as a basis for the various tests of hypothesis. The results indicate that for high degrees of clustering (25% and 10% levels) virtually all the whole-map statistics in table 3 would detect clustering [see table 6, where high or low counts (depending on the test statistic) are indicative of clustering]. At the 5% level some of the whole-map pattern detectors start to fail and below the 2.5% level nothing is found. This result is perhaps not too surprising, because with 5% clustering, only 43 (that is, 5% of the original 851 leukaemias) are point-source located. At the 2% clustering level only 16 cancers are assumed to be clustered, and only 8 at the 1% level. The whole-map blob statistics in table 7(a) suggest a similar result, although the point of failure is now moved below the 2.5% clustering level. The blob vicinity analysis reported in table 7(b) is similar. Here the counts are based on blobs in the 499 random data sets that overlap to some degree the observed data blobs. There is of course no distributional information to go with tables 6 and 7, although it could be generated by simulation; nevertheless, the blob results do appear quite useful. Moreover, the absence of type 2 errors is reassuring and has been supported by larger numbers of simulations.

A closer examination of the blob-specific results suggest that whereas clustering for the urban site is easily spotted down to about the 2% level, the rural cluster is not much in evidence. This result is hardly surprising because the data sets contain no additional cancers anywhere near the selected location below the 5% level. Indeed, the largest number of excess cancers ever assigned to the rural cluster source is 2. So again it is hardly surprising that it could not be detected.

Figure 1(a) shows a map of the blobs for the 2.5% clustering level. This map is extremely educational. There are 5 large blobs, some of which might readily be attributed as plausible interpretations had the data been real and not synthetic. The only blob that is significant is that shown in the middle right of the map which is based around the point source of the Gateshead cluster [see figure 1(b)]. The remainder are not even significant at the 25% level; yet the map patterns seem so real! The original GAM minimised this problem by using a very small threshold probability for the mapping. Here a much larger value is used

Table 6. Whole-map statistics for synthetic data: number of times out of 499 simulations that greater values are found than for the observed data.

Statistic	Degree of clustering in data (%)					
	25	10	5	2.5	2	1
Number of blobs	499	447	257	413	95	190
Number of circles after deduplication	0	0	24	48	362	30
Number of cancers in circles	0	0	2	4	447	55
Number of at-risk population in circles	0	0	2	4	464	73
Ink per cancer	499	498	486	483	87	370
Ink per at-risk population	494	492	487	484	47	361
Total ink used	0	0	9	41	394	83
Mean circle cancer rate in a blob	5	77	51	364	134	211
Mean circles per blob	0	0	29	40	404	72
Mean cancers per blob	0	0	3	7	451	76
Mean at-risk population per blob	0	0	3	6	464	92
Mean cancers per blob circle	0	0	15	28	418	104
Mean at-risk population per blob	0	0	2	6	478	117
Mean at-risk population per blob circle	9	3	3	8	478	132
Mean cancer rate per blob circle	499	497	431	463	86	415
Smallest Poisson probability within blob circle	499	499	422	456	231	360

Note: values above 475 or below 25 would indicate significance at about the 5% level (assuming a 1-tail test); it is left to the reader to figure out to which tail of the distribution each test statistic relates.

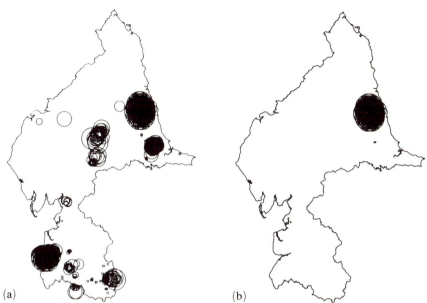

(a)   (b)

Figure 1. (a) Synthetic random data with cluster, (b) the only significant blob in figure 1(a).

Table 7. Blob statistics for synthetic data.

Statistic	Degree of clustering in data (%)					
	25	10	5	2.5	2	1
(a) Whole-map comparisons						
Number of circles after deduplication	499	499	497	473	4	0
Total number of cancers	499	499	497	494	10	0
Total excess at-risk population	499	499	496	489	23	0
Total at-risk population	499	499	497	495	1	0
Total ink used	499	499	497	461	0	0
Cancer rate	0	56	397	383	0	0
Smallest Poisson probability for any circle	499	499	422	456	51	0
Largest excess at-risk population	499	499	496	476	24	0
Total number of significant blobs found	1	1	1	0	0	0
(b) Comparisons restricted to overlapping blobs (vicinity analysis)						
Number of circles after deduplication	499	499	499	487	37	0
Total number of cancers	499	499	499	489	32	0
Total excess at-risk population	499	499	496	490	40	0
Total at-risk population	499	499	499	489	29	0
Total ink used	499	499	499	485	62	5
Cancer rate	499	335	477	465	19	0
Smallest Poisson probability for any circle	499	499	484	484	31	66
Largest excess at-risk population	499	499	496	483	30	0
Total number of significant blobs found	1	1	1	0	0	0

(p = 0.05) to avoid losing power in the hope that the blob analysis might remove the spurious results. Table 7 would indicate that on this occasion at least it did in fact work extremely well. Further simulation work has shown that this was not a chance result.

4.3 Results from the real data

The results from the synthetic data are mainly useful as a guide to which of the table 3 and table 4 test statistics are most likely to be sensitive measures of clustering. The cancer data used here come from the Northern and North West England Child Cancer Registries and relate to the period 1968–85. This source gives data on children aged 0–15 years who were diagnosed as having acute lymphoblastic leukaemia. These data are thought to be extremely accurate from a diagnosis point of view although their geographical precision is considerably poorer. The locational information is based on the postcodes of addresses at the time of diagnosis. These unit postcodes were then aggregated to census enumeration districts to ensure that all the data were represented by the same set of areal units; the alternatives would be to disaggregate the child counts from the census to unit postcodes, to use a mixture of postcode and census enumeration districts, or to aggregate everything to census enumeration districts. The population at risk is assumed to be children aged 0–15 years, counts of which are only available for 1971 and 1981 census enumeration districts. There are about 16 000 enumeration districts but with different boundary locations in each census. One of the major generic difficulties in this type of data set concerns the lack of annual information on the small area population at risk. The child population changed from a total of 1 761 290 in 1971 to 1 466 499 in 1981 and these changes may well cause major problems when trying to estimate the cancer rate for small areas. Some studies have used weighted estimates of population based on 1971–81 data but it is not clear as to whether this offers any real advantage. A better strategy might be to use a simulation to investigate these 'population-at-risk' effects or to subdivide the time period to reduce the magnitude of these problems.

In the computer runs performed here, 6 age–sex covariates (0–4, 5–9, 10–14) were used to remove the well-known age–sex differences in leukaemia incidence rates; although in fact it makes little difference to the GAM results. It would also be possible to allow for geographic differences in incidence rates for each age–sex group, although this has not been done here as there is no a priori basis for doing so. A variety of time periods are used: 1968–85 on a 1971 child count basis, 1968–85 on a 1981 basis, 1968–76 on a 1971 basis, and 1977–85 on a 1981 basis. The purpose is to identify any major effects that might be attributed to the use of different data on the population at risk.

One complete set of blobs is shown in figure 2(a) for the 1968–85 period in which 1981 child population counts were used. However, as in figure 1(a), many of these blobs possess a much smaller level of statistical significance than their map representation may imply. In table 8(a) and

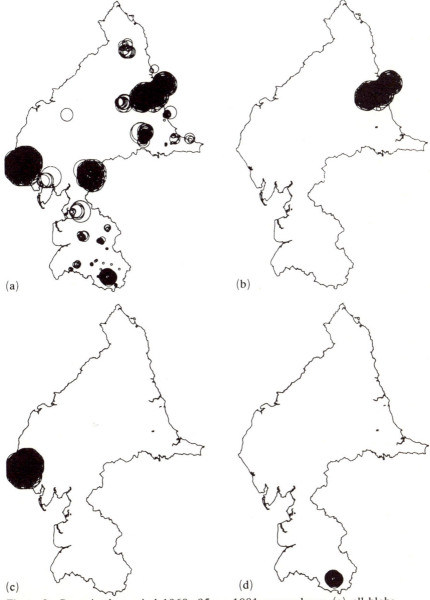

(a)   (b)

(c)   (d)

Figure 2. Cases in the period 1968–85 on 1981 census base: (a) all blobs, (b) blob 30, (c) blob 20, and (d) blob 3.

8(b) only blob 30 seems at all interesting; this is displayed in figure 2(b). The other two blobs (20 and 3) are shown in figures 2(c) and 2(d) and appear much less interesting from a descriptive inference point of view. These blob results may be compared with the whole-map statistics shown in table 9 which generally fail to detect any clustering. These results would appear to demonstrate the sensitivity of the blob-based vicinity analysis in identifying localised clustering. Whether this interpretation is justified depends on further simulation but the results look very promising.

When a subset of the data are used (for the period 1977–85) then only 1 blob appears at all interesting (see figure 3). The situation for the 1971-based data is different in that now there is more evidence of clustering at the whole-map level and less at the blob level. The exception is shown in figure 4(c), where a cluster is sufficiently strong to survive a different base population even though the cases on which it is based are probably closer to the 1981 census than to 1971. However, although many of these blob assessments are not of sufficient statistical significance to excite interest, the map patterns remain tantalisingly interpretable [see

Table 8. Blob statistics for leukaemia data.

Statistic	1971 base			1981 base					
	1968–85			1968–76		1968–85			1977–85
'Blob number'	21	22	27	10	12	3	20	30	23
(a) Whole-map comparisons									
Number of circles	301	119	162	87	115	32	340	483	470
Total number of cancers	106	86	318	26	20	249	132	490	481
Total excess of at-risk population	333	93	209	56	61	118	374	483	465
Total at-risk population	20	73	347	5	0	305	21	492	487
Total ink used	419	83	110	81	233	35	434	464	435
Cancer rate	0	0	340	0	0	392	0	310	348
Smallest Poisson probability	492	169	1	153	129	78	496	353	298
Largest excess of at-risk population	3	18	297	0	0	476	8	485	477
(b) Comparisons restricted to overlapping blobs (vicinity analysis)									
Number of circles	46	320	417	63	30	255	44	497	456
Total number of cancers	46	314	440	52	28	282	42	497	458
Total excess of at-risk population	46	316	420	60	29	271	44	497	456
Total at-risk population	45	314	445	41	25	286	42	497	459
Total ink used	46	312	419	61	31	270	44	495	454
Cancer rate	27	273	438	23	12	302	29	464	437
Smallest Poisson probability	46	328	304	73	31	272	44	476	436
Largest excess of at-risk population	46	30	429	35	14	317	41	497	458

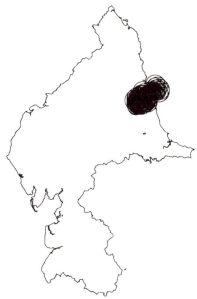

Figure 3. Cases in the period 1977–85 on 1981 census base: blob 23.

Table 9. Whole-map statistics for leukaemia data: number of times out of the 499 simulations that greater values were found than for the observed data.

Statistic	1971 base		1981 base	
	1968–85	1968–76	1968–85	1977–85
Number of blobs	148	71	126	51
Number of circles after deduplication	47	288	9	56
Number of cancers in circles	146	434	5	30
Number of at-risk population in circles	160	459	6	23
Ink per cancer	134	3	395	439
Ink per at-risk population	175	5	438	470
Total ink used	53	209	9	72
Mean circle cancer rate in a blob	174	133	93	154
Mean circles per blob	119	363	40	162
Mean cancers per blob	187	446	21	70
Mean at-risk population per blob	195	463	17	50
Mean cancers per blob circle	116	270	26	146
Mean at-risk population per blob	271	496	22	24
Mean at-risk population per blob circle	260	489	20	18
Mean cancer rate per blob circle	358	117	411	300
Smallest Poisson probability within circle in a blob	492	153	496	439
Number of blobs	41	34	42	34

for example, figures 5(b), 4(a), and 4(b)]. Maybe there is a danger in being too statistical and by so doing ignoring evidence. On the other hand, the results in figures 1(a) and 1(b) demonstrate the dangers of being too dependent on map patterns.

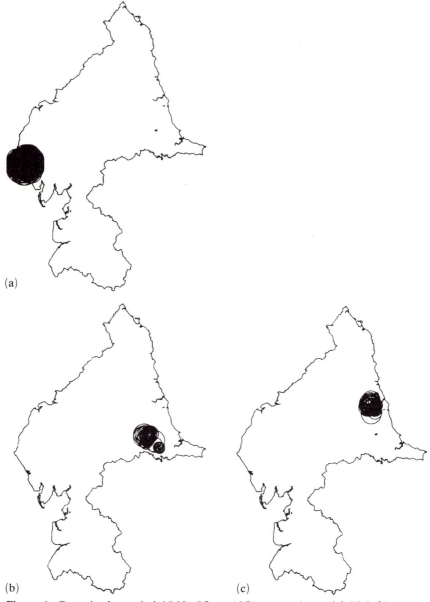

(a)

(b)   (c)

Figure 4. Cases in the period 1968–85 on 1971 census base: (a) blob 21, (b) blob 22, and (c) blob 27.

The next step will be to run other members of the GAM family on the same data and to compare the results.

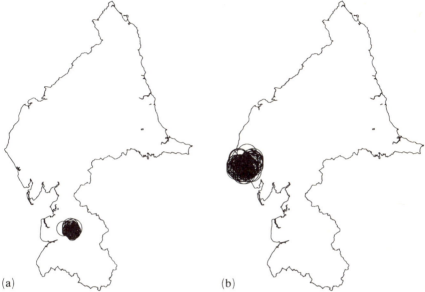

(a)   (b)

Figure 5. Cases in the period 1968–76 on 1971 census base: (a) blob 10 and (b) blob 12.

5 Conclusions

The aim in seeking to automate the analysis of spatial pattern is to develop a machine or analytical engine culture in which computer power is used to compensate for the lack of prior knowledge and theories about the nature of the processes responsible for the map patterns of interest. Of course it is easy to regard such ambition as little more than 'data trawling' in search of results, but it is difficult to see what alternatives could offer a more satisfactory approach to the problem being addressed here and being created in many other areas by the GIS revolution. The belief is expressed that the problems associated with a GAM-like comprehensive strategy for spatial pattern exploration can be overcome and that useful rather than dubious results can be obtained. It is, however, important not to underestimate the 'political', academic, and methodological problems that any attempt to create a machine-based analysis technology in areas where the concept is alien tends to produce. It is not an easy option and it runs counter to the prevailing wisdom about how statistical analysis on spatial data should be performed; however, this does not mean that such methods are necessarily doomed to fail.

To this end, I have described in this paper recent developments that have arisen from attempts to perfect an automated approach to the detection of cancer clusters. It is argued that the rudimentary, mark 1, geographical analysis machine does work. Some very striking patterns have been identified that appear to be real rather than due to chance. However, the original GAM/1 results almost certainly include some spurious clusters and the task is how best to identify the real ones and how to further the technology in the light of the various methodological problems that have been identified. The family of GAM(g, m, s) variants that now exist provide an integrated and flexible response to this problem, and the use of vicinity analysis and blob statistics represent another. An alternative use is worth considering; this would involve abandoning all notions that the GAM represents a statistical procedure and to regard it simply as a purely descriptive method, the role of which is merely to identify hypotheses for others to investigate at a more detailed scale. Indeed, maybe it is a major strategic error to view the GAM only from a narrow statistical perspective and then to strive to overcome the various hurdles that this brings. Maybe, the original view of the GAM as presenting a largely poststatistical procedure might be better for all concerned.

Nevertheless, the development of the GAM has served to emphasise the existence and importance of a whole string of interesting methodological problems that are endemic to many areas of spatial analysis. These tend to be difficult problems and it is too early to claim that they can all be solved. This combined with the imperfect nature of the available geographic information suggests that real-world applications should always proceed with care, with an emphasis on the conditional nature of the results and on the principle of caveat emptor. It is also necessary to be aware of the limitations of an exploratory style of study. All the GAM will do is to provide evidence that clustering exists; whether it is due to socioeconomic, demographic, or migration effects should be discounted prior to any search for potential environmental causes. However, there is no need to be too pessimistic, and the next few years could be very interesting indeed.

Acknowledgements. The author wishes to thank an everlengthening list of people who have directly and indirectly contributed to this work. The data came from the two cancer registries supported by the North of England Children's Cancer Research Fund and Cancer Research Campaign. Part of the GAM work was supported by the Economic and Social Research Council through their northeast Regional Research Laboratory at the University of Newcastle upon Tyne and by providing time on the Cray X-MP/48 supercomputer at the Rutherford Laboratory. The GAM/2 research was performed largely in a joint project with British Nuclear Fuels Limited and the United Kingdom Atomic Energy Authority on their Cray 2 supercomputer. Thanks are also due to Julian Besag, James Newell, David Appleton, Martin Charlton, and Chris Brunsdon for many stimulating and at times lively discussions. Finally, mention must be made of Alan Craft who started the whole GAM business by identifying the right question to ask in the first place.

References

Alexander F, Black R, Cuzick J, Edwards R, Openshaw S, Urquhart J, Ricketts J, Catwright R, 1989, "Tests for spatial clustering of rare disease: a comparative study", copy available from author

Besag J, Newell J, 1990, "The detection of clusters in rare diseases", forthcoming

Black D, 1984 *Investigation of the Possible Increased Incidence of Cancer in West Cumbria* report of the Independent Advisory Group (HMSO, London)

Clayton D, Kaldor J, 1987, "Empirical Bayes estimates of age-standardized relative risks for use in disease mapping" *Biometrics* **43** 671–681

COMARE, 1988 *Second Report* Committee on Medical Aspects of Radiation in the Environment (HMSO, London)

Cook-Mozaffari P J, Ashwood F L, Vincent T, Foreman D, Alderson M, 1987 *Studies in Medical and Population Subjects Number 51: Cancer Incidence and Mortality in the Vicinity of Nuclear Installations, England and Wales, 1959–80* (HMSO, London)

Cuzick J, Edwards R, 1990, "Tests for spatial clustering of events for inhomogenous populations" *Journal of the Royal Statistical Society, Series B* **57** 73–104

Davies J M, Inskip H, 1986 *Epidemiological Studies of General Population Groups Exposed to Low-level Radiation* (OECD, Paris)

Kinlen L, 1988, "Evidence for an infective cause of childhood leukaemia: comparison of a Scottish new town with nuclear reprocessing sites in Britain" *Lancet* **ii** 1323–1327

Kinlen L, 1989, "The relevance of population mixing to the aetiology of childhood leukaemia", in *Medical Response to Effects of Ionising Radiation* Eds W A Crosbie, J H Gittus (Elsevier, London) pp 272–278

Knox E G, 1964, "The detection of space–time interactions" *Applied Statistics* **13** 25–29

NRHA, 1989, "Review of the issue of apparent clusters of childhood leukaemia in the Northern Region: statement by an expert committee", Northern Region Health Authority, unpublished report, available from NRHA, Benfield Road, Newcastle upon Tyne NE6 4PY

Openshaw S, Craft A, 1989, "Some recent developments of the geographical analysis machine concept", in *Methodology of Enquiries into Disease Clustering* Ed. P Elliot (Small Area Health Statistics Unit, London) pp 35–38

Openshaw S, Charlton M, Craft A W, 1988a, "Searching for leukaemia clusters using a geographical analysis machine" *Papers of the Regional Science Association* **64** 95–106

Openshaw S, Charlton M, Craft A W, Birch J M, 1988b, "Investigations of leukaemia clusters by the use of a geographical analysis machine" *Lancet* **i** 272–273

Openshaw S, Charlton M, Cross A E, 1990, "Building a prototype geographical correlates exploration machine", forthcoming in *International Journal of GIS*

Openshaw S, Charlton M, Wymer C, Craft A W, 1987, "A mark I geographical analysis machine for the automated analysis of point data sets" *International Journal of Geographic Information Systems* **1** 335–358

Openshaw S, Wilkie D, Binks K, Wakeford R, Gerrard M H, Croasdale M R, 1989, "A method of detecting spatial clustering of a disease", in *Medical Response to Effects of Ionising Radiation* Eds W A Crosbie, J H Gittus (Elsevier, London) pp 295–308

Stone R A, 1988, "Investigation of excess environmental risk around putative sources: statistical problems and a proposed test" *Statistics in Medicine* **7** 649–660

Urquhart J, Black R, Buist E, 1989, "Exploring small area methods", in *Methodology of Enquiries into Disease Clustering* Ed. P Elliot (Small Area Health Statistics Unit, London) pp 41 – 49

Wakeford R, Binks K, Wilkie D, 1989, "Childhood leukaemia and nuclear installations" *Journal of the Royal Statistical Society, Series A* **152** 1 – 26

Wilkie D, 1986, "Outline planning application for a European demonstration fast reactor reprocessing plant at Dounreay, Caithness; public inquiry, days 72 – 74", transcript of proceedings; copy available from author

Some Problems in the Interpretation of Childhood Leukaemia Clusters

R WAKEFORD
British Nuclear Fuels plc, Risley

1 Introduction

The broadcasting of the television documentary "Windscale—the nuclear laundry" in November 1983 has led to a resurgence of interest in the distribution of the 'noninfectious' diseases, such as the leukaemias. In the television programme it was claimed that an unusually high number of leukaemias and other cancers had occurred in the young people living to the south of the Sellafield nuclear establishment on the West Cumbrian coast, and that the incidence rate of childhood leukaemias in the nearby village of Seascale was particularly unusual. Given the potential association of radioactive discharges with a high local incidence of cancer, the government set up the Independent Advisory Group (IAG) to examine the evidence and to make recommendations. The report of this group was published in July 1984 (IAG, 1984). It found that the claims concerning the number of cancers in the area were, in general, correct, but could find no obvious scientific explanation. In particular, the radiological evidence did not indicate a causal association with radioactive discharges. A number of recommendations for further epidemiological and radiological work were made, particularly in relation to the incidence rate of childhood leukaemias in Seascale.

Since 1984 other studies of cancer incidence and/or mortality in the vicinity of nuclear installations in the United Kingdom have been published, and the Committee on Medical Aspects of Radiation in the Environment (COMARE) has been established to examine the whole question of radiation-induced health effects in those nonoccupationally exposed. At present, it seems to be reasonably clear that a generally elevated incidence and/or mortality rate of leukaemias, and perhaps lymphomas, exists in the young people living in the neighbourhood of (certain) nuclear installations (COMARE, 1988; 1989; Cook-Mozaffari et al, 1987; 1989b; Forman et al, 1987; Wakeford et al, 1989a). What is not clear is whether the operations at these nuclear installations are directly responsible for these excess cases and/or deaths.

Radiological assessments continue to indicate that radiation exposures due to effluent discharges are far too low to account for the observed excesses (COMARE, 1989; Stather et al, 1988; Wheldon, 1989), and recent work has demonstrated that nonradiological mechanisms may be responsible. For example, Kinlen (1988; 1989) has shown that unusual population mixing may elevate the risk of childhood leukaemias, and Cook-Mozaffari et al (1989a) have shown that the pattern of cancer mortality rates in the vicinity of *potential* nuclear power station sites is similar to that around existing installations.

Regardless of the actual results obtained from the individual studies, this area of epidemiological research has highlighted a number of questions concerning the quality of the data, the appropriateness of the methodology, and the correctness of the inferences, adopted in these various studies. The answers to these questions can affect results and their interpretation, and in this paper I shall examine a number of the issues which have arisen.

2 Quality of data

The epidemiologist usually has a choice as to whether to employ cancer registration data for an analysis of cancer incidence, death certificate data for an analysis of cancer mortality, or both. This choice is particularly pointed in the study of childhood leukaemias because great advances have been made in the methods of treatment since 1960, with the result that more than 50% of children survive diseases that before this date were almost invariably fatal. Therefore, during the past 3 decades, mortality from childhood leukaemias has declined, even though the incidence of childhood leukaemias may not have. If treatment success during this period was geographically nonuniform, then spatial inhomogeneity of deaths amongst the population of children could be just a reflection of treatment regimes rather than a reflection of the pattern of incidence. There can be little doubt that definitive studies of the geographical distribution of the childhood leukaemias should be based upon incidence rather than mortality data.

However, the use of routinely available incidence data is not straight-forward. Historical data on cancer incidence are incomplete (Swerdlow, 1986) and spatial inhomogeneity of cancer registrations could be just a reflection of local registration efficiencies rather than a reflection of the pattern of incidence. For example, the raised registration rates of childhood cancers in the vicinity of the Atomic Weapons Establishment, Aldermaston, during 1971–80 are not, in general, evident as proportionally raised rates of mortality from childhood cancers (Wakeford, 1988). This presents difficulties of interpretation, as a high registration efficiency could, at least in part, be 'responsible' for the apparently high level of incidence. In this particular case, further work has shown that an especially high registration efficiency in the area is unlikely to be the explanation for the raised level of incidence (Draper et al, 1989). Nevertheless, this example illustrates the interpretational problem posed by this effect.

Cook-Mozaffari et al (1987) analysed both registration and mortality data in a comprehensive study of cancer incidence and mortality around 15 nuclear installations in England and Wales during the period 1959–80. These authors found substantial differences between the levels of cancer incidence and cancer mortality in the vicinity of nuclear installations, and concluded that registration data have a high relative completeness in these areas. As a consequence, Forman et al (1987), in a paper summarising the results of Cook-Mozaffari et al (1987), employed cancer mortality data only, arguing that cancer registration efficiency is too variable to allow registration data to be used with any confidence. The use of mortality data clearly presents other difficulties, but Cook-Mozaffari et al (1987; 1989b) have developed methods of analysis which they hope will reduce the effect of geographically variable medical practice and data quality.

Consequently, experience with the use of cancer registration and mortality data in the analysis of cancer incidence and mortality in the neighbourhood of nuclear installations in Britain has shown the need for care when employing historical data, and also the desirability of developing a complete and national scheme for cancer registration (COMARE, 1989).

Obviously, those analysing the incidence of cancer near nuclear sites should avoid the temptation of 'filling in' cases which are known to have been missed from the national or regional data bases, otherwise data capture in the area of interest can be enhanced to a level above that of the comparison area, possibly leading to spurious results. Special searches for cases in the vicinity of Sellafield certainly led to difficulties of interpretation of the early reports of high numbers of cancer cases (IAG, 1984).

A related issue is that of the uniformity of diagnostic and recording practices. The grouping of different types of leukaemia, which may have different aetiologies, hampers the epidemiological search for causes, and the use of such a grouping prior to 1968 does limit the general use of early data (Cook-Mozaffari et al, 1989b). A change in diagnostic conventions can introduce data bias, and this appears to be a particular problem in the distinction between some forms of childhood lymphoid leukaemia and some forms of childhood non-Hodgkin's lymphoma (COMARE, 1988). The possible variability of diagnostic criteria has to be borne in mind when analysing data.

Last, the generation of incidence or mortality rates in a geographical (or population-based) study requires a knowledge of the population at risk in a particular area. Population data are based upon the decennial national census, and upon estimates of what occurred in the intercensus years. Not only will a falling birth rate generally reduce the number of children at risk in a given area, but also migration from the inner-city areas during the 1970s can produce a drastic change in the number of children living within the centre of a conurbation between 1971 and 1981. If such population changes are not adequately dealt with, then an alarmingly high incidence or mortality rate could be artificially produced by, say, the use of 1981 census data with registration or mortality data for a time interval which includes a period prior to inner-city clearance.

What the recent studies of childhood leukaemia around nuclear sites have done is to reemphasise the importance of obtaining and using high-quality data, and of being aware of the problems which can arise in the use of historical registration and mortality data, and in the use of generally available population data.

3 Statistical methodology
For the proper interpretation of the results of an epidemiological study, it is necessary to distinguish between the hypothesis-generating study and the hypothesis-testing study (Davies and Inskip, 1986). In a hypothesis-generating study, data are, essentially, surveyed so that patterns of a possible causal nature are revealed. However, the geographical area(s) of interest will be defined by the nature of the distribution of the viewed data, and the boundaries which are used to quantify these selected patterns as, say, rates of incidence, may not have been specified in advance of the study. Consequently, any derived statistical significance is only nominal. This is because of the number of possible ways that the data could have been examined, and this number of possible comparisons must be taken into account in a proper assessment of statistical significance (Wakeford et al, 1989a). Under these circumstances, it is almost impossible to determine the statistical significance of any given pattern selected after the available data have been viewed, because the number of possible selections has not been determined.

This was one of the difficulties facing the Independent Advisory Group (IAG) in 1984 when confronted with the evidence for an unusually high rate of incidence of childhood leukaemias in the village of Seascale near Sellafield. The television team had not visited Sellafield with the intention of investigating any unusual health effects in the population living around the establishment, but had acted upon anecdotal reports once in the area. Thus, although over 3 decades the incidence rate of leukaemia in children under 10 years old in Seascale was calculated to be 10 times the national average (based on 5 cases), the effects of chance could not be ruled out or quantified because of the manner in which these particular data had been identified and then presented as an incidence rate. Nevertheless, given the circumstances, it was correct that the cases should be investigated further.

The use of exploratory studies, such as the rather unconventional one carried out for the 1983 television documentary, is that possible causal mechanisms are suggested which may be formally tested by using other data. Thus, the seemingly 'obvious' explanation for the excess of childhood leukaemias in Seascale was some form of gross underestimation of the leukaemogenic risk owing to radionuclides in the Sellafield effluent. It would seem reasonable to investigate this possibility by using data from areas around other nuclear facilities, or data from the Sellafield area gathered after the data as used by the IAG (1984), although caution is advisable because other, functionally different, installations have quantitatively and qualitatively different discharge records, and the

Sellafield discharge record is temporally very nonuniform, with levels being lowered substantially in recent years. However, from the point of view of statistical inference, the test of an hypothesis allows the effects of chance under the null hypothesis to be quantified, and this is clearly important (Wakeford et al, 1989a); but it is essential that the data employed in a hypothesis-testing study are independent of the data which originally generated the hypothesis, and that the structure of the test is not influenced by prior knowledge of the data available. Any such influence is liable to lead to an overestimation of the statistical significance obtained from the test, because boundary selection has, to some extent, been driven by the data, and this has not been accounted for in the analysis.

Prior knowledge of the cancer registration data for the area around the Dounreay establishment in northeast Scotland does seem to have influenced the presentation of the results of an analysis of leukaemia incidence in the young in this particular area (COMARE, 1988). The rate of incidence for an area lying within 12.5 km of Dounreay during the period 1979–84 was reported to be 10 times the Scottish average (based on 5 cases), with a statistical significance of 'less than 0.001' (Heasman et al, 1986). Wakeford et al (1989b) attempted to deal with the prior knowledge of the Dounreay data through a simulation exercise, and suggested that the actual significance of the incidence rate around Dounreay should be nearer 0.015. It will be seen that this result is still significant (at the 0.05 level), although less so than suggested in the original report, and there are other reasons for believing that a genuinely raised rate of incidence of childhood leukaemia exists in the vicinity of Dounreay (COMARE, 1988). However, this example does illustrate the difficulties that prior knowledge can present to the researcher.

A further example of the influence of prior knowledge on a potential hypothesis-testing study is that of the analysis of the incidence of childhood leukaemia in the vicinity of the two Ministry of Defence establishments in West Berkshire (Roman et al, 1987). In another television documentary, shown in 1985, it was suggested that leukaemia and lymphoma incidence in the young around the Aldermaston and, in particular, Burghfield establishments was abnormally high. Roman et al (1987), who had already been studying the incidence of childhood leukaemia in West Berkshire prior to the television programme, later confirmed the excess of cases, which was essentially confined to an excess of leukaemia cases in the under-5-year olds living within 10 km of the Burghfield facility. It is the inclusion of the Burghfield area that complicates the interpretation of this result. The Burghfield facility handles only manufactured weapons components and, as a consequence, radioactive discharges are comparable with those of hospitals, research institutes, and other industrial establishments in the area (COMARE, 1989). Cook-Mozaffari et al (1987) excluded Burghfield from their analyses for this reason, arguing that this level of discharge was considerably lower than those of the major nuclear installations. However, it would not have been easy for Roman et al to have followed the same course of action, given the interest generated by the television documentary. As a result, it is difficult to assess the significance of the Aldermaston and Burghfield analysis as a hypothesis-testing study, given the status of the inclusion of Burghfield within the study.

Consequently, the problems of 'multiple choice' and 'moving of goal-posts'—the simultaneous examination of many rates and the adjustment of boundaries on the basis of viewed data—should be studiously avoided in hypothesis-testing studies, otherwise serious problems of interpretation can follow, possibly to an extent which produces a 'significant' result that is purely an artefact of the statistical methodology.

An analysis structure which is driven by a knowledge of the available data usually favours 'false positive' results. On the other hand, the lack of statistical power in a study favours 'false negative' results. The statistical power of a study is the ability to detect a genuine effect, and depends upon the quantity of data used and the statistical methodology. Power considerations are especially pertinent to the study of childhood leukaemias in the vicinity of nuclear installations because the incidence of uncommon diseases in a rural, sometimes remote, area is under examination. Under such circumstances, it is unlikely there will be a large expected number of cases, and so appropriate methods, such as the pooling of data from a number of sites to increase the statistical power of a study, have to be considered. When expected numbers are small, failure to reject the null hypothesis must be interpreted with care because of lack of power, and the calculation of confidence intervals often provides valuable information, because small expected numbers—and hence low statistical power— produce relatively wide confidence intervals (Wakeford, 1989; Wakeford et al, 1989a). Power considerations provide a further reason for the use of data on the incidence of childhood leukaemias rather than on mortality, as incidence data generally generate larger expected numbers.

Certain other, sometimes unavoidable, effects can also weaken the statistical power of a study. One such effect is that of migration. The latent period between the initiation of a cancer and the clinical manifestation of the disease may be many years in length. Migration during latency would lead to the place of residence at diagnosis being different from that at which the possible exposure to some carcinogen occurred, thus reducing the sensitivity of a population-based study to geographically variable carcinogenic exposures. It is not easy to overcome this difficulty, although, for childhood cancers, place of residence at birth could be used instead of place of residence at diagnosis to investigate the effects of migration. Individual-based studies, such as birth cohort studies, may also be employed to deal with population migration. Migration after diagnosis will reduce the power of mortality studies relative to incidence studies, and if this migration is geographically nonuniform, because, say, some patients move to areas around treatment centres, then bias may be introduced.

The investigation of the power of a given statistical technique seems to have been a neglected area until comparatively recently, possibly because of the lack of computing facilities often required for simulation runs in such an investigation. When power studies have been carried out, it is sometimes found that standard methods have low power against particular nonrandom patterns (for example, Chen et al, 1984). My colleagues and I are examining the power of a χ^2 test which has been used by COMARE (1988) and Heasman et al (1987) to test for the departure of the recorded incidence of leukaemia in the young from a spatial Poisson process; and our (as yet unpublished) results suggest that this particular test has low power when compared with alternative techniques. Wartenberg and Greenberg (this volume) provide an interesting and useful discussion of the power of a number of statistical techniques often employed in the study of space–time clustering.

Not only should great care be taken in the construction of a study to ensure that methodological defects do not produce biased 'false positive' results, but also 'negative' results should be interpreted with caution because low power could mean that these results are compatible with a wide range of relative risks.

It should go without saying that any analysis of spatial patterns must be capable of quantitative interpretation for any meaningful conclusions on statistical significance to be drawn. One of the more elaborate, if not exotic, methods developed to investigate the spatial distribution of childhood leukaemia cases in the wake of the report of the IAG in 1984 was that of Openshaw et al (1988). The preliminary results of their method, although based upon population data from the 1981 census only and upon expected numbers which were not age–sex adjusted, did indicate visually unusual patterns of incidence of childhood lymphoid leukaemia in north and northwest England during the period 1968–85. However, it was not clear how these patterns might be properly quantified, or whether the 'strength' of a pattern which identified a particular excess of cases might be dependent upon the density of population surrounding that excess. Further work has removed the deficiencies in the calculation of expected numbers, and a methodology has been adopted which allows the statistical significance of a given excess of cases to be assessed, whilst retaining the spatial flexibility of the original method (Openshaw et al, 1989). This latest method does not reveal significant heterogeneity in the spatial distribution of lymphoid leukaemia cases amongst the children of north and northwest England during the period 1968–86, with the possible exception of the 4 cases in Seascale (Openshaw et al, 1990). It is unclear to me whether Openshaw (this volume) can further refine the original methodology of his earlier work

(Openshaw et al, 1988) to produce results which are amenable to
quantitative interpretation.

4 Confounding factors

A confounding factor is a covariable which correlates with the risk factor
of interest, and the control of confounders in the analysis of observational
data plays a major role in epidemiological methodology. Owing to the
possible presence of confounding factors, and because the causes of
most childhood leukaemia cases remain unknown (Doll, 1989), some
caution is necessary in the interpretation of excess cases of childhood
leukaemias. In addition, aetiological factors may be different for the
various types (and even subtypes) of childhood leukaemia, so that studies
in which all types of leukaemia are examined may not be appropriate
for the investigation of causal factors. However, as lymphoid leukaemia
accounts for 80% of the childhood cases of leukaemia, an excess of all
such cases will usually, but not necessarily, reflect an excess of cases of
lymphoid leukaemia. Nevertheless, it would be useful to distinguish
between the various forms of leukaemia in a study, if the data permit
(COMARE, 1988).

Nuclear installations are sited in rural, often remote, locations which
may possess levels of leukaemogenic risk factors which differ from those
in urban areas. Also, the construction and operation of a large industrial
facility will lead to a substantial influx of population into the surrounding
area. For example, the village of Seascale expanded rapidly in the late
1940s and during the 1950s to meet the employment demands of the
Sellafield site, and the village has contained a highly mobile, largely
young professional, population since that time. Kinlen (1988; 1989)
has shown that new towns in which population mixing has been particularly
marked have experienced a significantly raised rate of leukaemia mortality
amongst young children, and he has suggested that this could be due to
an enhancement of a rare leukaemogenic response to some infective agent.
The possibility that some of the excess cases of childhood leukaemia
near nuclear installations could be due to population mixing rather than
to the direct action of the installations has to be considered.

If major leukaemogenic risk factors have an appreciable geographical
variability then it is possible that the resulting spatial heterogeneity of the
distribution of cases of, or of deaths from, childhood leukaemia could
be detected. Spatial overdispersion of young deaths caused by lymphoid
leukaemia in the county districts of England and Wales during the period
1969 – 78 has been found by Cook-Mozaffari et al (1989b), although no
deviation from a Poisson distribution of cases of childhood lymphoid
leukaemia in north and northwest England during the period 1968 – 86
has been found by Openshaw et al (1990). It is possible that this
difference is owing to statistical power, and is being investigated by my
colleagues and me.

However, Cook-Mozaffari et al (1989b) found that, even after accounting for general spatial overdispersion, mortality amongst the young from lymphoid leukaemia was significantly raised in those districts near nuclear sites. Subsequently, Cook-Mozaffari et al (1989a) have investigated the level of cancer mortality around *potential* sites for nuclear power stations in England and Wales and have found a 'strikingly similar' pattern of deaths to that found around existing installations. The authors remark that areas near existing and potential sites might share unrecognised risk factors other than environmental radiation pollution. In this context, it is of interest that a marked excess of cases of childhood lymphoid leukaemia has occurred at Largo Bay in Scotland (Gerrard et al, 1986), and that this is also near a potential nuclear power station site.

That the raised levels of childhood leukaemia that generally exist near nuclear establishments might be due to the presence of some risk factor(s) other than the direct influence of the facility is suggested not only by the continued inability of radiological assessments to explain the excess cases in terms of radiation exposure from discharged material (Stather et al, 1988), but also by consideration of the nature and level of discharges from the various sites. Wheldon (1989) has noted that, although levels of discharge from nuclear sites vary substantially, the reported ratios of incidence of leukaemia in the young from areas around these sites do not reflect this marked variability. In addition, the radionuclides discharged from installations associated with excesses of childhood leukaemia cases vary from site to site and reflect the various functions of those installations (Berry, 1989; Taylor, 1989), so that it is unlikely that, say, exposure to plutonium is solely associated with the raised levels of incidence. However, it must be borne in mind that risk factors may not be directly associated with discharges, but still be related to site operations through some mechanism such as preconception germ cell injury in one or both parents while occupationally exposed to radiation or chemicals (Wheldon, 1989).

It is always tempting to interpret a statistical association as indicating a cause and effect relationship. One of the best known examples of an association which could be misleadingly interpreted as causation is the positive correlation between the numbers of storks and the numbers of humans (Hunter, 1981). Any Malthusian who went round killing storks on the basis of this association is liable to be disappointed. Similarly, although reductions in radioactive discharges might be considered desirable for other reasons, the impact on the risk of radiation-induced leukaemia could be very small.

5 Concluding remarks
The reported excess of childhood leukaemia cases in the village of Seascale has led to a flurry of radiological, epidemiological, and statistical activity (for example, *JRSS*, 1989). It does seem that an elevated risk of childhood

leukaemia exists near (certain) nuclear installations, although definitive
studies should be based upon the forthcoming national data base containing
details of the registrations of childhood cancer (COMARE, 1989).
However, radiological explanations have yet to be found (Stather et al,
1988), and nonradiological explanations may be required (Cook-Mozaffari
et al, 1989a; Kinlen, 1988; 1989).

Methodological advances have not been easy (*JRSS*, 1989), and the
low rate of incidence of the childhood leukaemias—about 35 cases per
million person-years—produces sparse data leading to low power,
particularly in lightly populated areas. However, some progress has
been made (for example, Bithell and Stone, 1989; Cook-Mozaffari et al,
1989b), and it will be interesting to watch future developments.

Finally, good methodology relies upon good data in order to arrive at
valid results. Hopefully, the national data base on childhood cancer
(COMARE, 1989) will provide the high-quality data required for definitive
analyses.

References
Berry R J, 1989, "Royal Statistical Society Meeting on Cancer near Nuclear
    Installations (contributed discussion)" *Journal of the Royal Statistical Society,
    Series A* **152** 377
Bithell J F, Stone R A, 1989, "On statistical methods for analysing the geographical
    distribution of cancer cases near nuclear installations" *Journal of Epidemiology
    and Community Health* **43** 79–85
Chen R, Mantel N, Klingberg M A, 1984, "A study of three techniques for
    time–space clustering in Hodgkin's disease" *Statistics in Medicine* **3** 173–184
COMARE, 1988 *Second Report* Committee on Medical Aspects of Radiation in
    the Environment (HMSO, London)
COMARE, 1989 *Third Report* Committee on Medical Aspects of Radiation in
    the Environment (HMSO, London)
Cook-Mozaffari P J, Ashwood F L, Vincent T, Forman D, Alderson M, 1987
    *Studies on Medical and Population Subjects 51: Cancer Incidence and Mortality in
    the Vicinity of Nuclear Installations, England and Wales, 1959–80* Office of
    Population Censuses and Surveys (HMSO, London)
Cook-Mozaffari P, Darby S, Doll R, 1989a, "Cancer near potential sites of
    nuclear installations" *Lancet* **ii** 1145–1147
Cook-Mozaffari P J, Darby S C, Doll R, Forman D, Hermon C, Pike M C,
    Vincent T, 1989b, "Geographical variation in mortality from leukaemia and
    other cancers in England and Wales in relation to proximity to nuclear
    installations, 1969–78" *British Journal of Cancer* **59** 476–485
Davies J M, Inskip H, 1986 *Epidemiological Studies of General Population Groups
    Exposed to Low-level Radiation* (OECD, Paris)
Doll R, 1989, "The epidemiology of childhood leukaemia" *The Journal of the
    Royal Statistical Society, Series A* **152** 341–351
Draper G J, Bower B D, Darby S C, Doll R, 1989, "Completeness of registration
    of childhood leukaemia near nuclear installations and elsewhere in the Oxford
    region" *British Medical Journal* **299** 952
Forman D, Cook-Mozaffari P, Darby S, Darby G, Stratton I, Doll R, Pike M,
    1987, "Cancer near nuclear installations" *Nature* **329** 499–505

Gerrard M, Eden O B, Stiller C A, 1986, "Variations in incidence of childhood leukaemia in South East Scotland (1970–1984)" *Leukaemia Research* **10** 561–564

Heasman M A, Kemp I W, Urquhart J D, Black R, 1986, "Childhood leukaemia in Northern Scotland" *Lancet* **i** 266, 385

Heasman M A, Urquhart J D, Black R J, Kemp I W, Glass S, Gray M, 1987, "Leukaemia in young persons in Scotland: a study of its geographical distribution and relationship to nuclear installations" *Health Bulletin* **45** 147–151

Hunter W G, 1981, "Six statistical tales" *Statistician* **30** 107–117

IAG, 1984 *Investigation of the Possible Increased Incidence of Cancer in West Cumbria* Independent Advisory Group (HMSO, London)

JRSS, 1989, "Royal Statistical Society Meeting on Cancer Near Nuclear Installations" *Journal of the Royal Statistical Society, Series A* **152** 305–384

Kinlen L, 1988, "Evidence for an infective cause of childhood leukaemia: comparison of a Scottish new town with nuclear reprocessing sites in Britain" *Lancet* **ii** 1323–1326

Kinlen L, 1989, "The relevance of population mixing to the aetiology of childhood leukaemia", in *Medical Response to Effects of Ionising Radiation* Eds W A Crosbie, J H Gittus (Elsevier, London) pp 272–278

Openshaw S, Charlton M, Craft A W, Birch J M, 1988, "Investigation of leukaemia clusters by use of a geographical analysis machine" *Lancet* **i** 272–273

Openshaw S, Wilkie D, Binks K, Wakeford R, Gerrard M H, Croasdale M R, 1989, "A method of detecting spatial clustering of disease", in *Medical Response to Effects of Ionising Radiation* Eds W A Crosbie, J H Gittus (Elsevier, London) pp 295–308

Openshaw S, Wilkie D, Binks K, Wakeford R, Gerrard M H, Croasdale M R, 1990, "The spatial distribution of childhood acute lymphoblastic leukaemia cases in the Northern and North-Western Regions of England during 1968–1986", in *Nuclear Energy* forthcoming

Roman E, Beral V, Carpenter L, Watson A, Barton C, Ryder H, Aston D L, 1987, "Childhood leukaemia in West Berkshire and Basingstoke and North Hampshire District Health Authorities in relation to nuclear installations in the vicinity" *British Medical Journal* **294** 597–602

Stather J W, Clarke R H, Duncan K P, 1988, "The risk of childhood leukaemia near nuclear establishments", report NRPB-R215 (HMSO, London)

Swerdlow A J, 1986, "Cancer registration in England and Wales: some aspects relevant to interpretation of the data" *Journal of the Royal Statistical Society, Series A* **149** 146–160

Taylor R H, 1989, "Royal Statistical Society Meeting on Cancer near Nuclear Installations (contributed discussion)" *Journal of the Royal Statistical Society, Series A* **152** 382

Wakeford R, 1988, "Childhood leukaemia incidence around nuclear installations" *Lancet* **i** 309

Wakeford R, 1989, "Infective cause of childhood leukaemia" *Lancet* **i** 331

Wakeford R, Binks K, Wilkie D, 1989a, "Childhood leukaemia and nuclear installations" *Journal of the Royal Statistical Society, Series A* **152** 61–86

Wakeford R, Dhodakia R, Binks K, Wilkie D, 1989b, "Leukaemia 'clusters' and nuclear installations with special reference to Dounreay", in *Radiation Protection—Theory and Practice* Ed. E P Goldfinch (IOP Publishing, Bristol) pp 75–78

Wheldon T E, 1989, "The assessment of risk of radiation-induced childhood leukaemia in the vicinity of nuclear installations" *Journal of the Royal Statistical Society, Series A* **152** 327–339

Part 2

Forecasting and Control

Epidemic Control and Critical Community Size: Spatial Aspects of Eliminating Communicable Diseases in Human Populations

A D CLIFF
University of Cambridge
P HAGGETT
University of Bristol

1 Introduction

The late 1970s were remarkable years in the world's epidemiological history. One major pandemic ended; another began. October 1977 saw the global eradication of one of mankind's great plagues when the last naturally occurring case of smallpox was tracked down in Somalia. Then, within 2 years, in the summer of 1979, the first official diagnosis in the United States of America of a patient with acquired immuno-deficiency syndrome (AIDS) signalled the start of a new global scourge.

Both events triggered renewed interest in disease eradication and the methods by which epidemics may be contained. Most of the new papers in this field over the last decade focus upon vaccine research and are clinically (or laboratory) related. However, as we have discussed before (Cliff and Haggett, 1989), many communicable disease have features which can be exploited to enhance the possibility of containing their spread geographically. In this paper we focus upon one such feature, namely the circumstances under which a disease ceases to be endemic and becomes epidemic, and we consider how this fracturing of the disease record in time may be exploited for spatial control purposes. To limit the size of the paper, we concentrate primarily upon the problems posed by the control of epidemic viral diseases of humans.

2 Types of control

A simple model of the spread of an infection through a population is shown in figure 1(a). The population at risk (susceptibles) of size S is added to by births at some rate γ. Infection proceeds by the mixing of the infected population of size I with the susceptible population; β is the mixing coefficient. Infectives recover at a rate μ. The total number of cases at time $t+1$ is then, at its simplest, an account of new cases less losses by recovery; that is,

$$I_{t+1} = I_t + \beta SI - \mu I. \tag{1}$$

As shown in figure 1(b), protection against infection can take place at two stages. Method A is to interrupt the mixing of infectives and susceptibles with protective spatial barriers. This may take the form of isolating an individual or community or by restricting the geographical

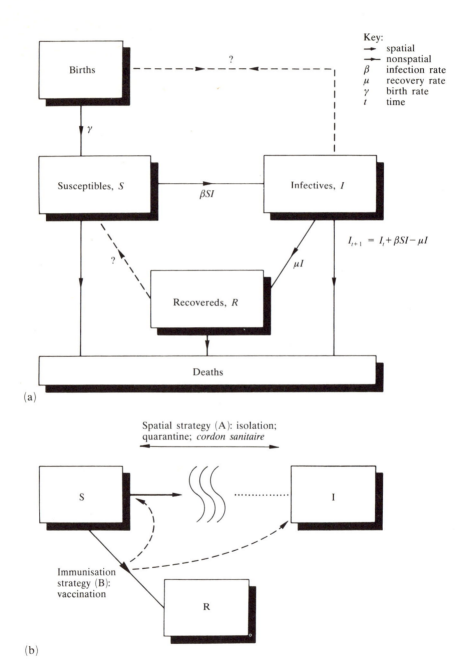

(a)

(b)

Figure 1. (a) A simplified model of an infectious process; (b) spatial (A) and nonspatial (B) intervention strategies to block the spread of infection. Source: Cliff and Haggett, 1989, page 317.

movements of infected individuals by quarantine requirements; another approach is by locating populations in supposedly 'safe' areas (Frenkel and Western, 1988). A third, largely theoretical possibility for human populations is the creation of a *cordon sanitaire* by the wholesale evacuation of areas. Alternatively, method B, shown in figure 1(b) may be employed. The route from 'susceptibles' to 'recovereds' is short-circuited by the establishment of immunity through some variant of immunisation.

Some of the spatial control strategies implied by the intervention points of methods A and B given in figure 1(b) are illustrated schematically in figure 2. In each of the four maps, infected areas are stippled and disease-free areas are left blank. *Local elimination* is, at first sight, apparently nonspatial in that the emphasis is on breaking the disease chain by vaccination. However, as May and Anderson (1984) show, the vaccination programme may itself have a geographical component. *Defensive isolation* is the building of a spatial barrier around a disease-free area by the use of, for example, vaccination or quarantine so that infectious cases are prevented from gaining access to the susceptible population at risk. *Offensive containment* is the reverse of the second case in that the spread of an outbreak within a disease-free area is halted and progressively eliminated by a combination of vaccination and isolation techniques. Last, *global eradication* describes the combination of the previous three methods; infected areas are progressively reduced in size and eventually eliminated on a worldwide basis. In this strictly global sense, eradication has been achieved in the case of only one virus

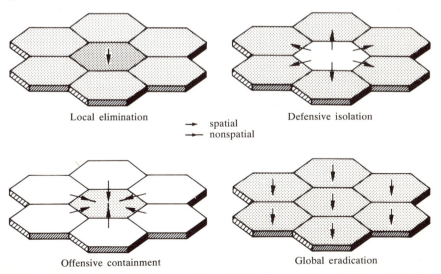

Figure 2. Four types of spatial control methods for epidemics. Source: Cliff and Haggett, 1989, page 318.

disease, smallpox (see the definitive account by Fenner et al, 1988). Local, national, or even continentwide elimination is different in kind in that reinvasion from reservoir areas can and does appear and that protective measures need to be maintained in the cleared areas.

Thus it is evident that local elimination is the key to global eradication. Once local disease-free areas are created, the aim must be to keep these free of disease by defensive isolation and offensive containment. Gradually, the cleared areas are extended to coalesce, and repetition of this basic process produces elimination in increasingly large geographical areas.

Given the crucial role of local elimination in the route to global eradication of a disease, we focus upon this aspect of the control problem in the remainder of the paper.

3 Local elimination of infection
To understand local elimination of an infectious disease, it is important to look first at the ways in which temporal and spatial breaks in disease chains occur naturally. From such models, the impact of intervention through immunisation methods such as vaccination can be more clearly appreciated.

3.1 Natural breaks in infection
The survival of the causative agent of an infectious disease to produce a continuous record of sickness is, inter alia, a function of the size of the population in which it is present. For the disease to be endemic, enough individuals at risk (susceptibles) must be present at all times for the chain of transmission of the agent from individual to individual to remain unbroken (Cliff et al, 1986).

The critical community size required to sustain endemicity has been studied in detail for measles in two classic papers, by Bartlett (1957) and by Black (1966). As shown in figure 3(a), Bartlett plotted the mean period (time interval) between epidemics (in weeks) for a sample of 19 English towns. This recurrence interval was found to be inversely related to the population size of the community, although in a nonlinear way. Given the reporting rates for measles at the time, from figure 3(a) it can be inferred that a population of around 250 000 is required to ensure continuous transmission chains.

Black extended Bartlett's work by examining the relationship between measles endemicity and population size in 18 island communities. Black plotted, on logarithmic scales, the percentage of months with notified cases against population size; the population size with 100% of months reporting denotes the endemicity threshold [figure 3(b)]. Of the islands studied by Black, only Hawaii with a total population (then) of 550 000 displayed clear endemicity. Other islands close to Bartlett's 250 000 value just failed to display endemicity.

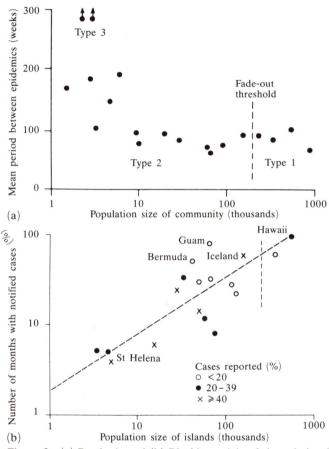

Figure 3. (a) Bartlett's and (b) Black's models of the relationship between epidemic frequency and population size. Source: Cliff et al, 1981, page 40.

3.2 Endemic threshold populations: theory

The basic notion of a threshold population, below which an infectious disease becomes naturally self-extinguishing, is paramount in articulating control strategies. It implies that vaccination may be employed to reduce the susceptible population below some critical mass so that biological processes may achieve the rest. As a result, attempts have been made to establish the endemicity thresholds for a variety of transmissible diseases. In table 1, we have summarised the findings for several diseases in relation to their *serial intervals*, where the 'serial interval' is defined as the average time between the observation of symptoms in one case and the observation of symptoms in a second case directly infected from the first. The table shows both the great variety in the population thresholds and the inverse relationship between the serial interval and the threshold population. But the large figure for influenza seems inherently unlikely since it begs the

historical paradox of how population densities were ever large enough
to allow the influenza virus to evolve and to be maintained; we will
return to this issue.

Once the population size of an area falls below the threshold then,
when the disease concerned is eventually extinguished, it can only recur
by reintroduction from other reservoir areas. Thus the generalised
persistence of disease implies geographical transmission between regions,
as shown in figure 4. Again, using measles as an example, we can see that
in large cities above the size threshold, like community A, a continuous
trickle of cases is reported. These provide the reservoir of infection
which sparks a major epidemic when the susceptible population, S,
builds up to a critical level. Since clinical measles confers subsequent
lifelong immunity to the disease, this buildup occurs only as children are
born, lose their mother-conferred immunity, and escape vaccination or
the disease. Eventually the S population will increase sufficiently for an
epidemic to occur. When this happens, the S population is diminished
and the stock of infectives, I, increases as individuals are transferred by
infection from the S to the I population. This generates the characteristic
'D'-shaped relationship over time between the sizes of the S and I
populations, as shown by the broken line on the end plane of the block
diagram (figure 4). If the total population of a community falls below
the 250 000 size threshold, as in settlements B and C of figure 4, measles
epidemics can, as we have noted above, only arise when the virus is
reintroduced by the influx of infected individuals (so-called index cases)
from reservoir areas. These movements are shown by the broad arrows
in figure 4. In such smaller communities, S is insufficient to maintain a
continuous record of infection. The disease dies out and S grows in the
absence of infection. Eventually S will become big enough to sustain an
epidemic when an index case arrives. Given that the total population of
the community is insufficient to renew S by births as rapidly as it is
diminished by infection, the epidemic will eventually die out.

It is the repetition of this basic process which generate the successive
epidemic waves witnessed in most communities. Of special significance

Table 1. The relationship between the infectious periods and minimum population
sizes required for endemicity of 5 communicable diseases.

Disease	Estimated infectious period (days)	Theoretical threshold population[a]
Hepatitis A	35	22 000 to 152 000
German measles	18	132 000
Whooping cough	~14	
Measles	12	300 000 to 500 000
Influenza	4	1 000 000 000

[a] Sources of values: Thacker, 1986; Yorke et al, 1979.

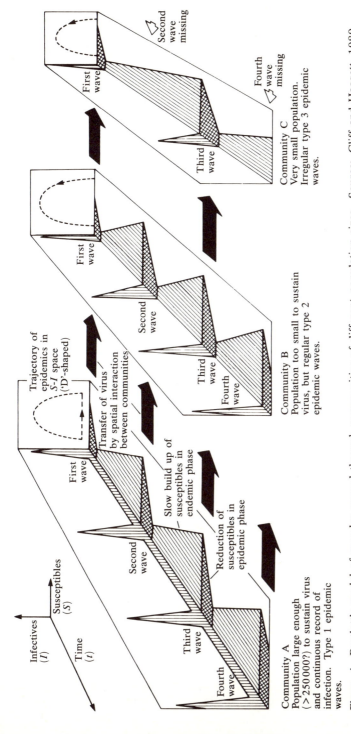

Figure 4. Bartlett's model of measles spread through communities of different population sizes. Source: Cliff and Haggett, 1989, page 322.

is the way in which the continuous infection and characteristically regular
type 1 epidemic waves of endemic communities break down as population
size diminishes into, first, discrete but regular type 2 waves in community B
and then, second, into discrete and irregularly spaced type 3 waves in
community C. Thus disease-free windows will automatically appear in
both time and space whenever population totals are small and geographical
densities are low.

Since S continues to grow by births in the absence of infection, very
large and sharply peaked epidemics can occur in small and isolated
communities if buildup takes place over a long period of time in the
absence of vaccination and index cases. Note also, in communities below
the population size threshold, that the base of the 'D'-shaped relationship
between the S and I populations is at zero with respect to I between
epidemics. This contrasts with communities like A where the nonzero
base reflects the continuous trickle of cases in the interepidemic phases.

3.3 Endemic threshold populations: empirical evidence
The extent to which the size and spacing of epidemics predicted by the
Bartlett model of figure 4 is observed in practice may be seen from
figure 5. In figure 5 the reported number of measles cases are plotted
as a time series for 4 countries arranged in decreasing order of population
size. The period covers 1945–70 and so is substantially prior to large-
scale vaccination. Figure 5(a) shows that, in the USA, with a population
of 210 000 000 in 1970, epidemic peaks arrived every year. In Britain,
with a 1970 population of 56 000 000, peaks occurred every 2 years.
Denmark [figure 5(c)], with a population of 5 000 000, had a more
complex pattern with some evidence of a three-year cycle in the latter
half of the period. Iceland (200 000) stands in contrast to the other
countries in that only 8 waves occurred in the 25-year period on an
approximate 4-year cycle, and no cases were reported in several years.

4 Icelandic evidence on critical community size
Critical community size is thus a central concept in the local elimination
of infection. If we can be sure of the population sizes below which
certain infectious diseases will become naturally self-extinguishing, local
elimination can be achieved by the reduction of the S population below
the appropriate threshold. This will replace blanket elimination as a goal
in control programmes, leaving natural processes to achieve the rest.

Given this crucial role for community size, the threshold populations
suggested in table 1 are now reexamined by using Icelandic data. The
checking of theoretical estimates against empirical data is made difficult
by different recording rates for particular diseases and by country-to-
country variations in reporting practices. Our work (Cliff et al, 1981)
on Icelandic data suggests that this country has especially accurate records,
and we use these data here to provide further empirical information

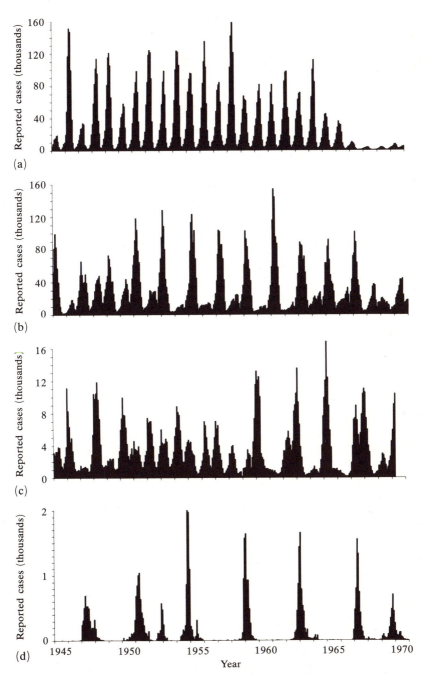

Figure 5. Reported cases of measles (monthly for the period 1945–70) for 4 countries arranged in descending order of population size: (a) USA, (b) United Kingdom, (c) Denmark, and (d) Iceland. Source: Cliff et al, 1981, page 39.

about critical population sizes for 4 of the diseases included in table 1:
German measles, whooping cough, measles, and influenza. In the case
of influenza, we note that Iceland's medical authorities, like those of
other countries which publish influenza morbidity data, record cases
without tying them to the particular virus type (A, B, or C).

In our method of analysis we follow Black (1966) and plot the
proportion of the 312 months between 1945 and 1970 in which the
disease was reported, in a geographically consistent set of 50 Icelandic
medical districts, against the population size of the districts. The end of
the period predates widespread vaccination against the diseases. The
results appear in figure 6. Fitting the regression lines shown in figure 6
enables the minimum population size threshold (that is, the population
at which cases of the disease will be first reported in all 312 months) to
be estimated by linear extrapolation. These thresholds are recorded in
table 2. The results for 3 of the diseases are broadly in line with the
findings of other workers. That for influenza appears to be uniquely
out of line, and yet simultaneously more plausible than the figure of
1 000 000 000 suggested by Yorke et al (1979).

The influenza virus is fundamentally different in its behaviour from
the others considered. The type A virus, which is responsible for most
epidemics and pandemics, changes its surface antigen characteristics
rather rapidly. The ability of the influenza virus to change by antigenic
shift and drift enables it to bypass population immunity conferred by

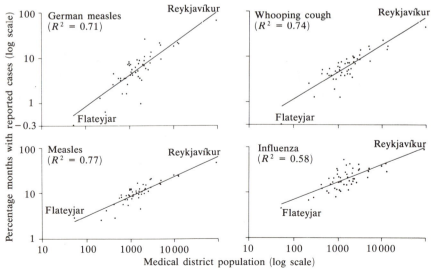

Figure 6. The relationship between percentage of months with reported cases of
4 communicable diseases in 50 Icelandic medical districts, January 1945 to
December 1970, and the average population size of the medical districts. Regression
lines can be used to estimate population thresholds for disease endemicity when
reported cases occur in all months. Source: Heilbrigðisskýrslur, 1945–70.

exposure to other influenza strains. As human immunity to influenza appears to be confined to a particular strain, this implies that the population of any community is recycled to provide a host for subsequent variants of influenza. This stands in contrast to measles and whooping cough where a single attack, because the causative agents are stable, confers lifelong immunity. Globally, there were 3 major shifts in the influenza virus in the period 1945–70 (0.115 shifts per year), and a much larger number of minor drifts. For example, Thacker (1986) reports 11 strains over a 17-year period (0.647 drifts per year).

To make the estimate of critical population size for endemic influenza directly comparable with other diseases shown in table 1 means a multiplier must be applied to the former. We calibrate the multiplier by dividing a population's expected life span (midperiod average 70.9 years for Iceland, 1945–70) by the number of different influenza strains to which it is exposed over its lifetime. For shifts, the multiplier is 70.9 years multiplied by 0.115 shifts per year (= 8.15); for drifts, it is 70.9 years multiplied by 0.647 drifts per year (= 45.87).

Application of the shift multiplier would raise the Icelandic estimate of the critical community size for influenza to the equivalent of nearly 1 000 000 (110 000 × 8.15 = 896 500) on a measles-comparable basis. Application of the drift multiplier would raise it to 5 000 000 (110 000 × 45.87 = 5 045 700). Although this brings the adjusted threshold into line with the sequence of estimates in table 1 based on the lengths of the infectious periods, it is still far short of the mammoth population size suggested by Yorke and others. For this latter gap to be bridged the population multiplier would need to be of the order of 10 000. This in its turn would imply a virus in an almost continuous process of change.

Much of the literature on the influenza A virus emphasizes the discrete two-step model of antigen change, with occasional large shifts associated with pandemics and minor drifts of greater frequency. However, when the cumulative probability distribution for influenza morbidity in Iceland (figure 7) is plotted as a recurrence interval (Gumbel, 1958), the plot

Table 2. Icelandic evidence on the minimum population sizes required for endemicity of 5 communicable diseases.

Disease	Estimated Icelandic threshold population[a]
Hepatitis A	not calculated[b]
German measles	98 000
Whooping cough	186 000
Measles	290 000
Influenza	110 000[c]

[a] Morbidity data from Heilbrigðisskýrslur, 1945–70.
[b] Data do not distinguish hepatitis A and B in the early part of the study period.
[c] 896 500 to 5 045 700, using drift and shift multipliers.

shows no clear-cut distinction between the two types. An equally plausible explanation of figure 7 would be to regard the severity of outbreaks as being on a continuum. Such a model would imply an unbroken hierarchy of antigen changes running from small and frequent to large and infrequent.

A continuum model would also go partway towards explaining some of the apparent anomalies in the observed behaviour of influenza. These include the difficulty of detecting a well-defined serial interval for the disease, apparently poor transmissibility within households, and multiple simultaneous outbreaks of the disease at widely separated geographical locations at the beginning of each influenza season. A continuum model would imply more minor subtypes in circulation than has been previously supposed, and thus more cases being independently generated rather than being the result of person-to-person transmission.

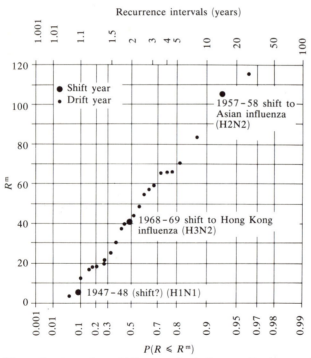

Figure 7. Annual morbidity rate for influenza, R^m (reported cases per thousand population), in Iceland, 1945–70, plotted as a Gumbel distribution to show the observed recurrence interval and the cumulative probability of obtaining an annual morbidity rate less than or equal to that shown on the vertical axis, $P(R \leqslant R^m)$. The recurrence interval is defined as $(1 + \text{number of years in the record})/(\text{rank of a given morbidity rate})$ where rank 1 is the highest rate and rank n is the lowest rate. The method is described in Gumbel (1958). An influenza year covers the period from 1 July until 30 June of the following year.

5 Impact of vaccination upon epidemic cycles

So far in this paper, we have concentrated upon establishing and testing the theoretical relationship between community size and probability of disease extinction in the absence of vaccination campaigns. Effective vaccines are now available for many infectious diseases (AIDS is an obvious exception) and vaccination either forms or will form the front-line method for reducing the S population below the critical community size for the disease. We therefore consider in this section the likely effect of vaccination campaigns. For illustrative purposes, we concentrate upon measles, the best understood of the diseases studied in this paper.

5.1 Theoretical considerations

The impact of partial vaccination policies upon the size and spacing of recurrent epidemics like those shown in figure 5 has been studied by Griffiths (1973), and by Anderson and Grenfell (1986). National campaigns to eliminate measles have generally aimed at a continued vaccination of about 90% of the susceptible population. Working with measles, Griffiths (1973) has used the Hamer–Soper and chain binomial models (Cliff et al, 1981, chapter 7) to examine the long-run effect upon a community of a continuing partial vaccination programme. If x denotes the proportion of children not artificially immunised by vaccination, Griffiths found that the critical community size for endemicity is multiplied by $1/x^2$. Thus 50% immunisation increases the critical community size from 250 000 to 1 000 000, and 90% immunisation increases the threshold to 25 000 000. Thus natural fade-out will become very widespread, enhancing the possibility of measles eradication. We have reviewed theoretical studies of immunisation strategies in an earlier paper (Cliff and Haggett, 1989).

5.2 Regional example: vaccination and measles cycles in the United States of America

Measles has long been recognised as a potentially serious disease. Its ability to spread rapidly through susceptible populations, especially in islands where the disease has been absent for many years, is well documented (Cliff et al, 1981). Although the illness is typically mild, serious complications of the respiratory tract, the middle ear, and central nervous system do occur and may result in death in malnourished populations. Thus in the developing countries, it has been estimated that 900 000 deaths occur annually as a result of measles infection. In the USA, in the early years of the 20th century, thousands of deaths were caused by measles each year (Hinman et al, 1980) and, at mid-century, an annual average of more than 500 000 measles cases and nearly 500 deaths were reported in the decade 1950–59.

It was against this background that the Centers for Disease Control, Atlanta, Georgia evolved, in the USA, a programme for the elimination of indigenous measles after a safe and effective vaccine was licensed for use in 1963 (Hinman et al, 1982). Work in Africa by McDonald, described in Hinman et al (1982), in the early 1960s led him to suggest that one way of reducing the population 'at risk' in large countries below this endemicity threshold would be to undertake an annual mass vaccination campaign reaching at least 90% of the susceptible children. By 1966, an epidemiological basis existed for the eradication of measles from the USA by using a programme with 4 tactical elements: (1) routine immunisation of infants at one year of age; (2) immunisation at school entry of children not previously immunised (catch-up immunisation); (3) surveillance; and (4) epidemic control (Senser et al, 1967). The immunisation target aimed for was 90% to 95% of the child population.

Following the announcement of possible measles eradication, considerable effort was put into mass programmes of measles immunisation throughout the USA. Federal funds were appropriated and, over the 3-year period 1966–68, an estimated 19 500 000 doses of vaccine were administered. The discontinuity that was induced in the time series of reported cases is shown for the USA as a whole in figure 8(a) and, for the Hawaiian Islands in figure 8(b). In 1962, the year before measles vaccine was introduced, there were 481 530 cases of measles reported in the USA. By 1966 this number had been reduced by more than 50% and by 1968 the reported incidence had plummeted to less than 5% of the 1962 level. In 1969 a vaccine against rubella (German measles) was licensed and all federal funds were targetted against rubella; no federal funds were allocated to the measles immunisation programme in the period 1969–71. As a result, measles vaccination in the public sector declined. The susceptible population rose and, as figures 8(a) and 8(b) show, the number of reported measles cases rose sharply, reaching 75 290 cases in 1971.

By the mid-1970s it was evident that the campaign against measles was running out of steam and that steady increases in measles incidence were occurring. To remedy this situation, a nationwide childhood immunisation initiative was launched in April 1977, followed by the announcement of a programme to eliminate indigenous measles from the USA by 1 October 1982. The immunisation goal aimed for was again 90% of the childhood population.

The impact of this second push against the disease is seen in the time series of figures 8(a) and 8(b), and the geographical effects were equally dramatic [figures 8(c) and 8(d)]. Figures 8(c) and 8(d) show, respectively, the distribution of counties in the USA which reported measles cases at the start of the campaign (1978) and 5 years later in 1983. The contraction of infection from most of the settled parts of the USA in 1978 to restricted areas of the Pacific Northwest, California, Florida, the Northeastern Seaboard, and parts of the Midwest is pronounced.

In 1983, 12 states and the District of Columbia reported no measles cases, and 26 states and the District of Columbia reported no indigenous cases. A total of 4 states (Indiana, 406 cases; Illinois, 216

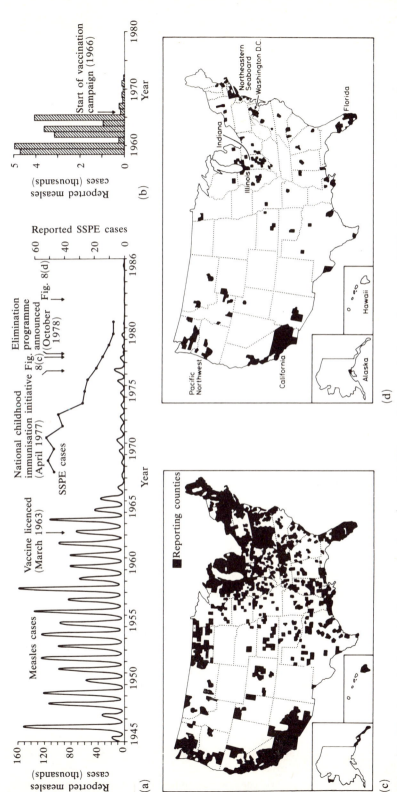

Figure 8. The impact of vaccination on measles waves: (a) US monthly reported measles cases, 1945–86, and subacute sclerosing panencephalitis (SSPE) cases, 1968–81; (b) reported measles cases in the Hawaiian Islands, 1959–80; (c) US counties reporting measles, 1978; and (d) US counties reporting measles, 1983. Source: Cliff and Haggett, 1989, page 325.

cases; California, 181 cases; Florida, 159 cases) accounted for 64% of the 1497 cases. Of the 3139 counties only 168 (5%) reported any measles cases. In contrast, measles was reported from 195 counties in 1982 and from 988 in 1978 when the measles elimination program began.

Unfortunately, total elimination still has not been achieved. Vaccination levels have fallen back since 1983 and the continued importation of measles cases from, primarily, Mexico and Canada has resulted in a resurgence of cases to 6216 in 1986. Nevertheless, the positive impact of the vaccination programme may be appreciated by examining the time-series incidence of an important although infrequent complication of measles infection, subacute sclerosing panencephalitis (SSPE).

SSPE is a slow-virus infection and is a degenerative neurological disorder characterised by the onset of mental deterioration and myoclonic seizures. It usually occurs late in childhood or in adolescence, approximately 7–10 years after acute measles illness. Although spontaneous improvement can occur, the vast majority of patients proceed over a period of months to years to generalised convulsions and eventually death. Although there is some dispute as to whether the SSPE visus is classical measles virus or a variant, it is generally agreed that it is a complication of severe measles attack and that measles vaccine is protective against it. The epidemiological evidence for the USA is shown in figure 8(a) where the number of reported SSPE cases is plotted for each year against the time series of reported measles cases. The decline in the reported SSPE cases has paralleled the decline in measles occurrence. In addition, studies by Halsey et al (1978) show from case-control studies that SSPE patients are less likely to have received measles vaccine than controls, and cohort analysis indicates that in the USA since 1966 there has been a progressive decrease in the incidence of SSPE in cohort groups born in succeeding years.

6 Conclusion

In this paper we have shown that, when considering worldwide eradication of any infectious disease as a theoretical goal, it is worth recalling that many are already periodically eliminated through natural processes in restricted geographical areas. Thus, it was the fact that measles cannot persist indefinitely in small, isolated communities that led Burnet and White (1972, page 17) to argue that "in principle vaccination against measles could allow eradication of measles from the globe".

Central to our understanding of periodic natural elimination of an infectious disease is the concept of critical community size. The threshold populations for natural elimination have been examined using Icelandic data for 4 diseases (German measles, whooping cough, measles, and influenza). For the first 3 of these, the results confirm existing theoretical work. In the case of influenza, the findings obtained are significantly different. A new model of the rate of antigenic drift and shift in the influenza virus has been proposed to account for the departures from existing theory. The differences also highlight the need for better models of the relationship between endemicity and population size than the essentially empirical approach implied in the Bartlett and Black methods. We are currently investigating this.

The main way in which populations susceptible to infectious disease are likely to be reduced below the relevant critical community size is by vaccination. Even when this is achieved, elimination is still an elusive goal. For example, in the case of measles, US experience shows that vigilant efforts to maintain high levels of vaccination, strong surveillance, and an aggresive response against imported cases in measles-free zones are still required to pin the disease back into diminishing areas.

The dramatic success of the WHO smallpox programme in eradicating smallpox (other than in laboratories) has inevitably raised the hope that other communicable diseases can also be eliminated. This view has been considered both for measles (Henderson, 1976; Hinman et al, 1980) and for poliomyelitis (Cvjetanovic et al, 1982; Stuart-Harris et al, 1982). Fenner et al pointed out that smallpox was well suited (perhaps uniquely well suited) to global eradication (1988, page 422). A detailed comparison of the characteristics of smallpox, both biological and socioeconomic, with measles and poliomyelitis showed only a partial overlap: measles shared 10 of the 14 smallpox characteristics but poliomyelitis only 5 (Fenner, 1986). Any immediate hope of global eradication of other diseases thus seems remote. But for measles, at least, a feasible scenario is that a greater number of developed countries will follow the lead of the USA and attempt to eliminate measles nationally as an endemic disease. Whether the coalescence of disease-free zones in developed countries would ever allow a sustained attack on measles reservoirs in developing countries will depend as much on politics and economics as on epidemiology. Any campaign will need to follow a spatial policy in which success in limited geographical areas is a prerequisite to any continentwide or global programmes.

References
Anderson R M, Grenfell B T, 1986, "Quantitative investigations of different vaccination policies for the control of congenital rubella syndrome (CRS) in the United Kingdom" *Journal of Hygiene* **96** 305–333
Bartlett M S, 1957, "Measles periodicity and community size" *Journal of the Royal Statistical Society A* **120** 48–70
Black F L, 1966, "Measles endemicity in insular populations: critical community size and its evolutionary implication" *Journal of Theoretical Biology* **11** 207–211
Burnet M, White D O, 1972 *Natural History of Infectious Disease* fourth edition (Cambridge University Press, Cambridge)
Cliff A D, Haggett P, 1989, "Spatial aspects of epidemic control" *Progress in Human Geography* **13** 315–347
Cliff A D, Haggett P, Ord J K, 1986 *Spatial Aspects of Influenza Epidemics* (Pion, London)

Cliff A D, Haggett P, Ord J K, Versey G R, 1981 *Spatial Diffusion: An Historical Geography of Epidemics in an Island Community* (Cambridge University Press, Cambridge)

Cvjetanovic B, Grab B, Dixon H, 1982, "Epidemiological models of poliomyelitis and measles and their application to the planning of immunization programmes" *Bulletin of the World Health Organization* **60** 405–422

Fenner F, 1986, "The eradication of infectious diseases" *South African Medical Journal: Festschrift Supplement* 11 October, pages 35–39

Fenner F, Henderson D A, Arita I, Jezek Z, Ladnyi I D, 1988 *Smallpox and Its Eradication* (World Health Organization, Geneva)

Frenkel S, Western J, 1988, "Pretext or prophylaxis? Racial segregation and malarial mosquitoes in a British tropical colony: Sierra Leone" *Annals of the Association of American Geographers* **78** 211–228

Griffiths D A, 1973, "The effects of measles vaccination on the incidence of measles in the community" *Journal of the Royal Statistical Society A* **136** 441–449

Gumbel E J, 1958, "Statistical theory of floods and droughts" *Journal of the Institution of Water Engineers* **12** 157–184

Halsey N A, Modlin J F, Jabbour J T, 1978, "Subacute sclerosing panencephalitis (SSPE): an epidemiological review", in *Persistent Viruses* Eds J G Stevens, G J Todoro, C F Fox (Academic Press, New York) pp 101–114

Heilbrigðisskýrslur, 1945–70, English translation: Public Health in Iceland (Office of the Director General of Public Health, Reykjavík, IS 101, Iceland)

Henderson D A, 1976, "Smallpox-eradication and measles-control programs in West and Central Africa" *Industry and Tropical Health* **6** 112–120

Hinman A R, Brandling-Bennett A D, Bernier R H, Kirby C D, Eddins D L, 1980, "Current features of measles in the United States: feasibility of measles elimination" *Epidemiologic Reviews* **2** 153–170

Hinman A R, Orenstein W A, Bloch A B, Bart K J, Eddins D L, Amler R W, Kirby C D, 1982, "Impact of measles in the United States", paper read at the International Symposium on Measles Immunization, Washington, DC; copy available from A R Hinman, Centers for Disease Control, Atlanta, GA

May R M, Anderson R M, 1984, "Spatial heterogeneity and the design of immunization programmes" *Mathematical Biosciences* **72** 83–111

Senser D J, Dull H B, Langmuir A D, 1967, "Epidemiological basis for the eradication of measles" *Public Health Report* **82** 253–256

Stuart-Harris C, Western K A, Chamberlayne E C (Eds), 1982, "Can infectious diseases be eradicated?" *Review of Infectious Diseases* **4** 912–984

Thacker S B, 1986, "The persistence of influenza A in human populations" *Epidemiologic Reviews* **8** 129–142

Yorke J A, Nathanson N, Pianigiani G, Martin J, 1979, "Seasonality and the requirements for perpetuation and eradication of viruses in populations" *American Journal of Epidemiology* **109** 103–123

Assessing the Impact of Some Spatial Representation Systems on the Forecasts of a Multiregion Disease Model

R W THOMAS
University of Manchester

1 Introduction

The capability to forecast the spread and timing of an epidemic enables the implementation of effective management strategies for both vaccination and control. However, the history of infectious disease modelling reveals that this task is complex, especially the prediction of spatial spread. The important contributions of Bartlett (1960) and Bailey (1975) emphasise predicting the temporal incidence of disease in closed communites, and the development of mathematical mechanisms to mimic different infectious aetiologies. For example, the state equations required to represent the behaviour of measles (Cliff et al, 1981) and influenza (Cliff et al, 1986), which spread by simple person-to-person contact, have been adapted successfully to cope with more intricate biologically vectored and carrier-borne diseases, like malaria and typhoid, respectively (Bailey, 1975). By comparison, the apparent dearth of rigorous mathematical analyses of disease incidence in space is explained by the difficulties of taking direct account of all the distances separating the individuals who form the susceptible and infective populations.

Instead, progress in forecasting space–time disease incidence has relied on the adoption of approximate approaches to space where, in a multiregion setting, its effects are represented by surrogate measures such as migration rates (Baroyan and Rvachev, 1967; Rvachev and Longini, 1985) or some form of gravity interaction (Murray and Cliff, 1977; Thomas, 1988a). In this paper I am concerned with the second of these measures and investigate how different forms of spatial interaction model impact upon the output of a multiregion disease model.

In the begining sections, I develop results presented in another paper (Thomas, 1990) and show how different ideas about spatial representation lead to the derivation of disease models which either contain infectivity rates specific to each region, or a single rate specific to the disease under study. The effect of these alternative representations is then tested by using a deterministic model calibrated to mimic the distribution of Hodgkin's disease over the regions of Greater Manchester. Simulation of these spatial formulations reveals some significant impacts on the timing of the predicted epidemic. It will be shown how it is useful to distinguish between effects which occur when the epidemic is 'in phase' amongst the regions, and effects when the regions are 'out of phase'.

2 Specifying a multiregion disease model for Hodgkin's disease

Hodgkin's disease (HD), a cancer of the body's lymphatic system, has
no proven infectious disease agent (Grufferman and Delzell, 1984).
However, some quite compelling evidence has accumulated to suggest
HD might well be transmissible and, therefore, fall within the ambit of
disease modelling strategies (Thomas, 1986). This evidence relies on
the bimodal age-specific incidence of HD, which is typified by an
unusual peak for a cancer among young adults (MacMahon, 1966) and
by examples of significant space–time clustering among case distributions
(Greenberg et al, 1983; Mangoud et al, 1985). The work reported here
is not designed to contribute to the controversy surrounding the possible
infectivity of HD (Smith and Pike, 1976). Instead, HD is chosen for
study because the evidence also suggests the mechanisms of its possible
transmission might be quite complex, which poses some interesting
problems for testing the properties of a disease model. In particular,
studies of the contact networks of HD cases (Vianna, 1975) are especially
relevant for modelling because they show that, if the transmission of the
disease is to be maintained, a healthy population of asymptomatic
carriers is required to complete the network.

Figure 1 presents a state diagram for a model of an 'infectious' HD
in a closed community (adapted from Thomas, 1986). The state
variables include a susceptible population, x, who may acquire the HD
agent from two possible sources: first, from contact with a member of
the carrier population, y; and, second, from an incubating infective, z,

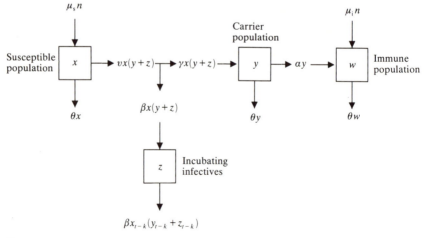

Key:
n total population v contact rate α rate of loss of infective power
μ_s birthrate, susceptibles γ carrier formation rate θ deathrate
μ_i birthrate, immune β diseased formation rate

Figure 1. Structure of the single-region HD model: variables and relations.

yet to develop symptoms of HD. The total population of the community is denoted by n, which is assumed to include an immune population who gain their status either through birth or as carriers who have ceased to be infective.

The remaining terms in figure 1 show the transactions between the state variables which are assumed to occur in each unit of time, dt. In this specification, infectivity is described by a set of parameters which control transactions from x to y and z. The term $x(y+z)$ represents the maximum number of contacts that could potentially occur in dt, and v is the disease contact rate measuring the proportion of all possible contacts that lead to transmission of the HD agent. This pool of infection serves as a source both for new carriers and for incubating infectives. Entry into the carrier sector is controlled by γ, the carrier formation rate, and incubating infectives are formed at a rate β. These rules imply $v = \gamma + \beta$, because the entire pool of new infectives must be transferred out of the susceptible sector.

Transactions out of the carrier population to the immune population are controlled by α, the rate at which carriers lose their power to infect. Incubating infectives are removed according to a constant incubation period, k, such that new cases entering at time $t - k$ will be removed at time t.

Entry to the susceptible population is controlled by the birthrate of susceptibles, μ_s, which is taken to be a constant fraction of the community birthrate, μ, and therefore applies to the total population, n. Last, a constant deathrate, θ, is applied to all but the incubating infective population where the removal of cases is equivalent to deaths. A more detailed justification of these assumptions as they apply to the evidence for an infective HD agent may be found in two previous papers (Thomas, 1986; 1988b).

To change this specification for a single community into a multiregion setting, the main population variables $(x, y, z, \text{ and } n)$ are subscripted to record their values in the $i \, (= 1, \dots, m)$ regions. Ideas from spatial interaction theory are now introduced to represent the spread of infection around the regions. The approach adopted here is to redefine the term for new infections, $vx(y+z)$, in the community specification such that the transfer of susceptibles to the carrier and incubating infective populations follows according to:

$$v_i x_i \sum_j^m (y_j + z_j) \exp(-\lambda d_{ij}) = \gamma_i x_i \sum_j^m (y_j + z_j) \exp(-\lambda d_{ij}) +$$

$$\beta_i x_i \sum_j^m (y_j + z_j) \exp(-\lambda d_{ij}), \qquad \forall i \,. \qquad (1)$$

In this way, the number of contacts between susceptibles resident in region i and all the infectives, $y_j + z_j$, resident in j will decay in accordance with the distance beween the regions, d_{ij}, following a negative exponential distribution with constant parameter λ. Notice the infectivity rates (v_i, γ_i and β_i) are subscripted to indicate that, for the moment, varying interpersonal contact rates are assumed for each region.

Given this specification, deterministic equations can be obtained by defining the differential coefficient which controls the change in the value of each variable as the difference between its inputs and outputs, which, for the multiregion HD model, leads to the set

$$\frac{\mathrm{d}x_i}{\mathrm{d}t} = \mu_s n_i - v_i x_i \sum_j^m (y_j + z_j)\exp(-\lambda d_{ij}) - \theta x_i, \qquad \forall i, \tag{2}$$

$$\frac{\mathrm{d}y_i}{\mathrm{d}t} = \gamma_i x_i \sum_j^m (y_j + z_j)\exp(-\lambda d_{ij}) - \alpha y_i - \theta y_i, \qquad \forall i, \tag{3}$$

and

$$\frac{\mathrm{d}z_i}{\mathrm{d}t} = \beta_i x_i \sum_j^m (y_j + z_j)\exp(-\lambda d_{ij})$$
$$- \beta_i x_{i,t-k} \sum_j^m (y_{j,t-k} + z_{j,t-k})\exp(-\lambda d_{ij}), \qquad \forall i. \tag{4}$$

3 Equilibrium conditions
Both the interpretation and the calibration of models derived from equations (2)–(4) rely on a knowledge of the equilibrium which arises when the differential coefficients are all set equal to zero. If the values of the parameters μ_s, θ, k, and α are assumed to be given, then the following procedures can be used to obtain equilibrium values ($x_i^{(0)}$, $y_i^{(0)}$, and $z_i^{(0)}$, $\forall i$) for the state variables.

Assume that the observed long-term average of diseased cases per unit of time, $\bar\eta$, in the study area is equivalent to the equilibrium number of new cases of HD, $\beta x^{(0)}(y^{(0)} + z^{(0)})$, then the corresponding averages for each region, $\bar\eta_i$, are obtained by multiplying $\bar\eta$ by n_i/n. In this calculation, the further assumption is made that the equilibrium arises when regional incidence of disease is in proportion to regional population. The equilibrium number of incubating cases, $z_i^{(0)}$, in each region is now defined as the accumulation of k (the incubation period) inputs of new cases, $\bar\eta_i$, which occur prior to their removal as 'deaths' from HD [see equation (4)]. This relationship provides the result

$$z_i^{(0)} = k\bar\eta_i, \qquad \forall i. \tag{5}$$

Let c denote an estimate of the long-term average number of carriers observed for each incubating case; then the equilibrium regional carrier populations will be given by

$$y_i^{(0)} = cz_i^{(0)}, \qquad \forall i. \tag{6}$$

Equilibrium values for the susceptible populations can now be obtained by manipulating the deterministic equations. Setting equations (2) and (3) to zero and redefining new carrier contacts [the term involving γ_i in equation (3)] as all new contacts [the term involving v_i in equation (2)] minus new diseased contacts, $\bar{\eta}_i$, we are led to the result

$$x_i^{(0)} = \frac{1}{\theta} [\mu_s n_i - \bar{\eta}_i - y_i^{(0)}(\alpha + \theta)], \qquad \forall i . \tag{7}$$

This expression is useful because the equilibrium values for the susceptible population can be calculated without prior knowledge of the infectivity rates and the exponential decay parameter. These properties rely on the existence of a second term invovling x_i in equation (2) in addition to the infectivity transaction. In this case the inclusion of the death term (that is, θx_i, $\forall i$) in the specification is responsible for this property.

4 Representation systems for the infectivity parameters
The most frequently encountered method of representing infectivity rates in the literature (Bailey, 1975; Murray and Cliff, 1977; Rvachev and Longini, 1985; Thomas, 1988a) is to allow them to vary in line with the regional populations. Such a representation is obtained from equation (4) by setting the output term equal to the observed average incidence of new cases in each region (that is, $\bar{\eta}_i$, $\forall i$) and rearranging to obtain

$$\beta_i = \bar{\eta}_i \left/ x_i^{(0)} \sum_j^m (y_j^{(0)} + z_j^{(0)}) \exp(-\lambda d_{ij}), \qquad \forall i . \right. \tag{8}$$

The regional variability of the β_is is attributable to the behaviour of the denominator in the right-hand side of equation (8), which counts the number of contacts involving susceptibles resident in region i. This count will only be in exact proportion with its respective $\bar{\eta}_i$, thereby generating identical β_is, for the exceptional case when all $\bar{\eta}_i$ are equal (that is, for a uniform distribution of population) and each region is equally accessible to all complementary regions. Any deviation from this ideal will cause disproportionality between the susceptible contacts and their respective η_is such that variable β_is are required to restore the equilibrium. The same properties apply to the other infectivity rates in the HD model which are obtained from the deterministic equations as

$$v_i = \frac{1}{x_i^{(0)}} (\mu_s n_i - \theta x_i^{(0)}) \sum_j^m (y_j^{(0)} + z_j^{(0)}) \exp(-\lambda d_{ij}), \qquad \forall i . \tag{9}$$

and

$$\gamma_i = v_i - \beta_i, \qquad \forall i . \tag{10}$$

In a discussion of a multiregion disease model based on migration, rather than spatial interaction principles, Bailey (1975, page 353) justifies this use of infectivity rates as balancing factors on the grounds that a single infectious individual living in a community 5 times larger than another, is unlikely to have an acquaintance circle also 5 times larger than the individual's from the smaller community. Thus infectivity rates vary to even out the effects of population distribution. However, this variability does not square with the epidemiological notion that, in a closed community, a disease will be characterised by a single infectivity rate, and it is possible to develop plausible multiregion models with this property.

The implication of equations (8)–(10) is that the region-specific rates vary around average rates for single study areas, given by

$$\beta = \bar{\eta} \left[\sum_i^m x_i^{(0)} \sum_j^m (y_j^{(0)} + z_j^{(0)}) \exp(-\lambda d_{ij}) \right]^{-1} , \qquad (11)$$

$$v = (\mu_s n - \theta x^{(0)}) \left[\sum_i^m x_i^{(0)} \sum_j^m (y_j^{(0)} + z_j^{(0)}) \exp(-\lambda d_{ij}) \right]^{-1} , \qquad (12)$$

and

$$\gamma = v - \beta . \qquad (13)$$

Clearly, if these single rates are introduced to the multiregion HD model then a scaling system, S, is needed to ensure that the susceptible contacts generate the observed average case incidence (that is, $\bar{\eta}_i$, $\forall i$). I will evaluate 2 approaches to this problem: S2, an adaption of the scaling system employed in the origin–destination constrained spatial interaction model in which the epidemic populations are adjusted to maintain equilibrium zonal contacts; and S3, the application of exponential decay parameters which are regionally variable. Because the 3 infectivity rates [equations (11)–(13)] are calculated from the same total of susceptible contacts, the scaling systems can be derived in terms of any one of them. In this instance β is used for simplicity of expression.

Let C_{ij} represent the number of contacts between susceptibles in i and infectives in j, and $\mathbf{C}^{(0)}$ denote the equilibrium contact matrix. This matrix will be symmetrical above and below the principal diagonal because the epidemic populations (that is, $x_i^{(0)}$, $y_i^{(0)}$, $z_i^{(0)}$, $\forall i$) are held in fixed proportions with their respective $\bar{\eta}_i$s. Consequently, an acceptable system of scaling must maintain this symmetry, otherwise it would be necessary to assume that susceptibles and infectives resident in the same region were subject to different levels of accessibility to the remainder of the study area.

The problem can now be stated as the need to find scalar values which generate $\mathbf{C}^{(0)}$ subject to the constraints

$$\sum_j^m C_{ij}^{(0)} = \frac{\bar{\eta}_i}{\beta} , \qquad \forall i . \qquad (14)$$

Thus the sum of the scaled contacts in each row and column of $\mathbf{C}^{(0)}$ must equal the expected number of contacts given by $\bar{\eta}_i/\beta$ [see equation (12)]. Adaption of the scaling system employed in the origin–destination constrained spatial interaction model leads to the following set of contacts:

$$C_{ij} = A_i x_i^{(0)} A_j (y_j^{(0)} + z_j^{(0)}) \exp(-\lambda d_{ij}), \qquad \forall i, j. \tag{15}$$

In fact, this formulation is simpler than that used in the standard interaction model because the symmetry required for the terms in $\mathbf{C}^{(0)}$ ensure that each row scalar, A_i, must be equal to its equivalent column scalar, $A_{j=i}$. These scalar values are found from the standard method of calculating the ratio between the expected number of contacts in region i, $\bar{\eta}_i/\beta$, and the corresponding unscaled contact totals, which yields

$$A_i = \frac{\bar{\eta}_i \beta^{-1}}{x_i^{(0)}} \sum_j^m A_j (y_j^{(0)} + z_j^{(0)}) \exp(-\lambda d_{ij}), \qquad \forall i, \tag{16}$$

and

$$A_j = \frac{\bar{\eta}_j \beta^{-1}}{y_j^{(0)} + z_j^{(0)}} \sum_i^m A_i x_i^{(0)} \exp(-\lambda d_{ij}), \qquad \forall j. \tag{17}$$

These equations are solved in the usual way by setting the A_js in equation (16) equal to unity to obtain first estimates for the A_is, and then repeatedly cross-substituting updated estimates until convergence is reached. These converged scalar values are measures of the inaccessibility of the epidemic populations of each zone to the population distribution over the entire study area. Thus we can make linear adjustments to these populations to restore the equilibrium contact totals, $\bar{\eta}_i/\beta$.

An alternative to weighting the epidemic populations, S2, is to scale by the introduction of regionally variable, exponential decay parameters (λ_i, $\forall i$, and λ_j, $\forall j$), which relaxes the assumption held so far that the propensity to make contacts of a given distance remains constant throughout the study area. This scaling system, S3, might be justified, for example, if it were established that peripheral regions experienced a higher proportion of contacts from outside the study region. Similarly, factors like a centralised distribution of employment, which are exogenous to the model design, might well enhance the propensity to travel from the periphery.

Formally, this scaling problem may be stated as finding the set of decay exponents which generate equilibrium regional contact totals from:

$$C_{ij}^{(0)} = x_i^{(0)} (y_j^{(0)} + z_j^{(0)}) \exp(-\lambda_i \lambda_j d_{ij}), \qquad \forall i, j, \tag{18}$$

such that the elements of $\mathbf{C}^{(0)}$ satisfy the constraints imposed by equations (14). Again, the symmetry required for $\mathbf{C}^{(0)}$ ensures each row exponent, λ_i, must equal its equivalent column exponent, $\lambda_{j=i}$.

The required values for the decay exponents are found by using standard optimisation procedures. Let successive iterations be denoted by K; then starting values for the decay exponents are obtained from the estimate chosen for the study region decay exponent, λ. If travel propensities are taken to be the same in each zone, then the relationship

$$\lambda_i \lambda_j = \lambda, \qquad \forall i, j, \tag{19}$$

will hold to provide starting values from

$$\lambda_i^K = \lambda_{j=i}^K = \lambda^{1/2}, \qquad K = 1, \forall i. \tag{20}$$

Substituting these values in equation (18) will provide us with our first estimates of the number of susceptible contacts originating in each region. Second estimates are obtained by comparing these contact totals with the equilibrium totals $(\bar{\eta}_i/\beta, \forall i)$, which yields

$$\lambda_i^K = \lambda_{j=1}^K = \lambda_i^{K-1} \frac{\beta}{\bar{\eta}_i} \sum_j^m C_{ij}^{(0), K-1}, \qquad K = 2, \forall i. \tag{21}$$

The linear interpolation used to obtain these second estimates is then repeated until a satisfactory convergence is achieved.

These scaling systems each lead to changes to the deterministic equations (2)–(4) that contain region-specific infectivity rates, and which will now be denoted by S1. For the system S2 the differential coefficient for the susceptible population is given by

$$\frac{\mathrm{d}x_i}{\mathrm{d}t} = \mu_s n_i - A_i x_i \sum_j^m A_j (y_j + z_j) \exp(-\lambda d_{ij}) - \theta x_i, \qquad \forall i. \tag{22}$$

With the system S3 in operation this coefficient becomes

$$\frac{\mathrm{d}x_i}{\mathrm{d}t} = \mu_s n_i - v x_i \sum_j^m (y_j + z_j) \exp(-\lambda_i \lambda_j d_{ij}) - \theta x_i, \qquad \forall i. \tag{23}$$

Similar rearrangements can be applied to obtain the coefficients for y and z that accompany S2 and S3.

The deterministic equations describing each scaling system are too complex to allow the derivation of analytical solutions which describe the exact behaviour of the state variables through time. However, an approximate understanding can be gained by writing each equation in difference form which, for the example of equation (23), leads to

$$x_{i, t+\Delta t} = x_{i, t} + [\mu_s n_i - v x_{i, t} \sum_j^m (y_{j, t} + z_{j, t}) \exp(-\lambda_i \lambda_j d_{ij}) - \theta x_{i, t}] \Delta t, \qquad \forall i. \tag{24}$$

This difference equation allows the susceptible population for S3 to be projected for successive times, t, by choosing appropriate starting values for $t = 0$, and a simulation interval, Δt. In the following, the simulations are calibrated from HD data for Greater Manchester, in which is recorded the monthly incidence from 1962–76 and, accordingly, $t = 1$ month and $\Delta t = 0.05$ months. This value of Δt requires the difference coefficients estimated for each month, $\Delta x_i/\Delta t$, $\Delta y_i/\Delta t$, etc, to be an aggregate of 20 individual interpolations. Experimentation with lower values of Δt showed that little increase in accuracy was achieved over the selected value, which suggests the numerical errors due to the use of linear equations such as equation (24) as approximations for their analytical equivalents are quite small.

An alternative to differencing is stochastic simulation in which the transactions in the deterministic equations are treated as transition probabilities. The variable output generated by stochastic methods makes them the more suitable for forecasting. However, the deterministic style is much more suited to unravelling the behaviour of different models where a single output simplifies the process of comparison.

5 Calibration procedures

The variety of models that have been described are calibrated by using data for the incidence of HD over a grid of $m = 16$ cells (each 64 km^2) covering the majority of the urban area of Greater Manchester (see figure 2). Moreover, the rates needed to solve the different versions of the HD model have been abstracted from a previous analysis (Thomas, 1988a) in which I fitted a stochastic version of the model to the monthly incidence of the disease in Greater Manchester for the period 1962–76. These fits were not globally optimum because of the presence of unknown parameter values. Instead, the fit relied on matching the observed periodicity of HD (59 months) with simulated periodicities obtained from hypothesised combinations of the susceptible birth rate, μ_s, the carrier removal rate, α, the incubation period, k, and the ratio of carriers to incubating infectives, c. The best fitting set amongst the combinations that were tested is listed in table 1. This set describes an equilibrium characterised by a low input of susceptible births, a high rate of carrier removal (all carriers are removed or die each month), a short incubation period ($k = 3$ months), and a ratio of carriers to incubating infectives (c) of 4.67. This last figure is taken from the contact networks of HD cases

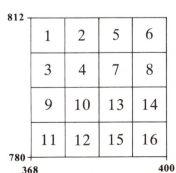

Figure 2. Locations (i, j) of the regions of Greater Manchester and their Ordnance Survey national grid references.

studied by Vianna (1975) in Albany (NY), and the incubation period is an estimate taken from an analysis of the space-time interaction of the Greater Manchester cases (Mangoud et al, 1985).

Most of the spatial terms in the models are calibrated by using results I have presented in another paper (Thomas, 1990). The interpretation

Table 1. The parameters and equilibrium values used for the simulations.

i	Epidemic populations[a]				Regional infectivity rates[a]		
	$x_i^{(0)}$	$y_i^{(0)}$	$z_i^{(0)}$	$\bar{\eta}_i$	v_i	γ_i	β_i
Terms derived from the distribution of the observed population							
1	334	3.78	0.81	0.27	0.00146	0.00136	0.00010
2	321	3.64	0.78	0.26	0.00099	0.00092	0.00007
3	210	2.38	0.51	0.17	0.00117	0.00109	0.00008
4	704	7.99	1.71	0.57	0.00066	0.00062	0.00004
5	371	4.20	0.90	0.30	0.00094	0.00088	0.00006
6	148	1.68	0.36	0.12	0.00140	0.00131	0.00009
7	914	10.36	2.22	0.74	0.00058	0.00054	0.00004
8	544	6.16	1.32	0.44	0.00086	0.00080	0.00006
9	148	1.68	0.36	0.12	0.00133	0.00124	0.00009
10	581	6.58	1.41	0.47	0.00070	0.00065	0.00005
11	37	0.42	0.09	0.03	0.00216	0.00202	0.00014
12	321	3.64	0.78	0.26	0.00113	0.00105	0.00008
13	951	10.78	2.31	0.77	0.00060	0.00056	0.00004
14	297	3.36	0.72	0.24	0.00095	0.00089	0.00006
15	383	4.34	0.93	0.31	0.00101	0.00094	0.00007
16	62	0.70	0.15	0.05	0.00166	0.00155	0.00011

v (total infectivity rate) = 0.00079
γ (carrier rate) = 0.00073
β (incubating case rate) = 0.00006

Terms derived from the distribution of a uniform population							
1	395	4.48	0.96	0.32	0.00137	0.00128	0.00009
2	395	4.48	0.96	0.32	0.00108	0.00101	0.00007
4	395	4.48	0.96	0.32	0.00085	0.00079	0.00006

Regions 6, 11, and 16 take the values of region 1; regions 3, 5, 8, 9, 12, 14, and 15 those of region 2; and regions 7, 10, and 13 those of region 4.
v (total infectivity rate) = 0.00106
γ (carrier rate) = 0.00099
β (incubating case rate) = 0.00007

Constant disease characteristics
μ_s (susceptible birth rate) = 0.000036
α (carrier removal rate) = 0.9986
θ (carrier death rate) = 0.0014
k (incubation period) = 3 months
c (carriers per incubating case) = 4.67
$\bar{\eta}$ (average number of HD cases per month in Greater Manchester) = 5.12

Constant spatial characteristics
p (external contact proportion) = 0.05
r (average radius of Greater Manchester) = 2.568×8 km
λ (exponential decay parameter) = 1.3275
$d_{i=j}$ (within-region travel distance, for all i) = 0.3971×8 km

[a] Persons per month.

of the exponential decay parameter, λ, is based on the following expression, which is adapted from Masser and Brown (1977):

$$\lambda = \frac{1}{r} \ln(p^{-1}) . \tag{25}$$

Here p is the proportion of all contacts estimated to be external to the study area, and r is the approximate radius of the area. In most of the simulations which follow, p is set arbitarily at 0.05 to give $\lambda = 1.3275$ (where $r = 2.2568$, in units of 8 km). However, also examined are cases where $p = 1$ (that is, $\lambda = 0$) such that all contacts take place irrespective of distance under homogeneous mixing, and $p = 0$ (so that $\lambda \to \infty$) where all contacts are internal and the mixing is heterogeneous.

The distances between the centres of the regions shown in figure 2 are expressed in units of 8 km—the side lengths of each square region. The within-region distances $(d_{i = j}, \forall i)$ are not directly measurable and have been given values according to a result given in Thomas (1990). Each $d_{i = j}$ is defined as the expected contact distance within region i, where contact distances are distributed according to a negative exponential distribution with a known decay parameter, λ. Moreover, this distribution is truncated so that the expected distance is calculated for contacts within the region which begin at the centre and do not cross its boundary. Assuming approximately circular regions with constant radii r_i (for all i), then the expected contact distance over each r_i, $\bar{d}(r_i)$, is obtained as:

$$\bar{d}(r_i) = \frac{1}{\lambda} [-\exp(-\lambda r_i)] = d_{i = j}, \qquad \forall i . \tag{26}$$

For Greater Manchester, the radius of every region is 0.5642×8 km, $\forall i$, such that with $\lambda = 1.3275$, the within-region distances, $\bar{d}(r_i)$, are obtained from equation (26) as 0.3971×8 km, $\forall i$.

Notice this estimate of the within-region distance depends on the exponential decay parameter such that, when $\lambda = 0$ (homogeneous mixing) $\bar{d}(r_i) = r_i$, and when $\lambda \to \infty$ (heterogeneous mixing) $\bar{d}(r_i) \to 0$. Thus the within-region distance is consistent only if the application of the model requires a single value of λ estimated from a known external contact probability, p. In cases where variations in the value of λ are to be explored, then $\bar{d}(r_i)$ must be fixed to the estimate of λ that is dependent on p; otherwise, the application would require the unwarranted assumption that λ is capable of transforming distance. In the results that follow, the fixed value of λ is taken to be 1.3275 ($p = 0.05$).

The equilibrium values of the epidemic populations $(x_i^{(0)}, y_i^{(0)}, z_i^{(0)}, \forall i)$ were generated by distributing the average monthly incidence of HD in Greater Manchester between 1962 and 1976 ($\bar{\eta} = 5.12$ cases) over the 16 regions in proportion to their populations to give the equilibrium regional incidences ($\bar{\eta}_i, \forall i$). Equations (5)–(7) were then used to calculate equilibrium values for the epidemic populations, and equations (8)–(13)

were used to calculate the infectivity rates required for the scaling systems S1–S3. These terms are listed in table 1, which also shows the equivalent values that would arise if the population of Greater Manchester were distributed uniformly over the 16 regions ($\bar{\eta}_i = 5.12/16, \forall i$).

Table 2. Effects of the exponential decay parameter on the regional rates and scalars.

i	Values based on a uniform distribution of population				
	v_i	$\sum C_{ij}^{(0),\,S1}$	A_i	λ_i	$\sum C_{ij}^{(0),\,S2+S3}$
$\lambda = 0$					
1	0.00014	34435	1.0000	0.0000	34435
2	0.00014	34435	1.0000	0.0000	34435

Values for regions 3–16 are the same as those for region 1 (or 2) except for the

$\lambda = 1.3275$					
1	0.00137	3505	1.2147	0.9718	4516
2	0.00108	4451	1.0128	1.1442	4516
3	0.00108	4451	1.0128	1.1442	4516
4	0.00085	5664	0.8390	1.3156	4516
5	0.00108	4451	1.0128	1.1442	4516
6	0.00137	3505	1.2147	0.9718	4516
7	0.00085	5664	0.8390	1.3156	4516
8	0.00108	4451	1.0128	1.1442	4516
9	0.00108	4451	1.0128	1.1442	4516
10	0.00085	5664	0.8390	1.3156	4516
11	0.00137	3505	1.2147	0.9718	4516
12	0.00108	4451	1.0128	1.1442	4516
13	0.00085	5664	0.8390	1.3156	4516
14	0.00108	4451	1.0128	1.1442	4516
15	0.00108	4451	1.0128	1.1442	4516
16	0.00137	3505	1.1247	0.9718	4516
$\lambda = 5.0000$					
1	0.01470	327	1.0267	2.2083	343
2	0.01400	343	1.0008	2.2354	343
3	0.01400	343	1.0008	2.2354	343
4	0.01330	361	0.9738	2.2606	343
5	0.01400	343	1.0008	2.2354	343
6	0.01470	327	1.0267	2.2083	343
7	0.01330	361	0.9738	2.2606	343
8	0.01400	343	1.0008	2.2354	343
9	0.01400	343	1.0008	2.2354	343
10	0.01331	361	0.9738	2.2606	343
11	0.01470	327	1.0267	2.2083	343
12	0.01400	343	1.0008	2.2354	343
13	0.01331	361	0.9738	2.2606	343
14	0.01400	343	1.0008	2.2354	343
15	0.01400	343	1.0008	2.2354	343
16	0.01470	327	1.0267	2.2083	343

Note: For the contact totals, $\sum C_{ij}^{(0),\,S1}$ and $\sum C_{ij}^{(0),\,S2+S3}$, the summation is made

6 Results

6.1 Spatial representation effects

The results listed in table 2 summarise how the representation systems S1–S3 respond to both the distribution of population and the degree of

Values based on the observed distribution of population				
v_i	$\sum C_{ij}^{(0),\,S1}$	A_i	λ_i	$\sum C_{ij}^{(0),\,S2+S3}$
0.00014	29054	1.0000	0.0000	29054
0.00014	27978	1.0000	0.0000	27978

contact totals based on the observed distribution of population.

0.00146	2772	1.5397	0.7832	5156
0.00099	3939	1.1804	1.0029	4965
0.00117	2179	1.3428	0.9145	3247
0.00066	12955	0.8649	1.3088	10886
0.00094	4792	1.1602	1.0269	5729
0.00140	1290	1.6312	0.8143	2292
0.00058	19072	0.7928	1.4178	14132
0.00086	7652	1.0875	1.0683	8403
0.00133	1351	1.5354	0.8568	2292
0.00070	10043	0.9108	1.2469	8976
0.00216	208	2.3481	0.6833	573
0.00113	3453	1.3219	0.9118	4970
0.00060	19250	0.8120	1.3919	14705
0.00095	3780	1.1973	1.0052	4584
0.00101	4613	1.2214	0.9700	5920
0.00166	453	1.9344	0.7547	955
0.01764	230	1.3558	1.9256	423
0.01616	242	1.3209	1.9753	407
0.02343	109	1.6186	1.7964	266
0.00788	1085	0.8982	2.3525	892
0.01438	322	1.2429	2.0312	469
0.03227	56	1.9474	1.5805	188
0.00613	1813	0.7885	2.4680	1158
0.01038	472	1.0412	2.2107	689
0.03282	55	1.9371	1.6215	188
0.00925	763	0.9807	2.2692	735
0.10030	4	3.7545	1.2163	47
0.01712	229	1.3469	1.9491	407
0.00601	1922	0.7794	2.4869	1205
0.01685	214	1.3729	1.9229	376
0.01414	329	1.2307	2.0389	485
0.06334	51	2.9262	1.3379	78

for $j = 1, \dots, m$.

mixing denoted by the exponential decay parameter. The results given for a uniform population were obtained by setting equilibrium regional caseloads $\bar{\eta}_i = \bar{\eta}/m$, $\forall i$, and then calibrating in the usual way.

The essential nature of the three representation systems is illustrated by the difference between the regional contact totals, $\sum C_{ij}^{(0)}$ ($j = 1, ... , m$), listed for S1 and those that accompany S2 and S3. Under S1 the contact totals are not subjected to scaling, whereas under S2 and S3 they are the equilibrium regional contacts, $\bar{\eta}_i/\beta$, achieved after the application of either of the two scaling systems. In this way, the contact totals for S1 are in proportion to those totals used for S2 and S3 according to the value of the ratio β_i/β, and also the equivalent ratio for the two other infectivity rates. Thus regions with a below-average infectivity rate, $\beta_i \leqslant \beta$, generate an above-average number of contacts, and vice versa when $\beta_i \geqslant \beta$. For example, comparison of the infectivity rate chosen for Greater Manchester ($v = 0.00079$, $\lambda = 1.3275$, see table 1) with the corresponding regional infectivity rates shows that only the accessible central regions (4, 7, 10, 13) generate above-average contact totals (table 2).

When a constant infectivity rate is assumed for the study area, the scalars A_i and λ_i, $\forall i$, adjust for differences in regional accessibility. Values for these scalars obtained under several assumptions are listed in table 2. Their variation is more difficult to explain than that in the infectivity rates, because each row scalar, A_i, works in conjunction with a set of column scalars, A_j, $\forall j$. With a few minor exceptions in rank order, the scalar values follow the same general pattern identified for the regional infectivity rates. Regions where $A_i < 1$ are characterised by above-average accessibility, and the value indicates the need to scale down the contact total and to assume a lower propensity to make contact. Conversely, values of $\lambda_i > \lambda^{1/2}$ indicate a lower propensity to travel long distances to compensate for the above-average accessibility.

The solutions listed in table 2 are designed to show how the scalars and infectivity rates respond to population distribution and the exponential decay parameter. With $\lambda = 0$ there is no distance-decay effect and the regional scalars all take their neutral values. Let λ be equal to 1.3275 with a uniform population, then the scalar values group into 3 classes to reflect variations in accessibility defined by the 3 total distances, $\sum d_{ij}$ ($j = 1, ... , m$; $\forall i$), that arise from the location of each region in a grid with 16 cells. Thus the central regions (4, 7, 10, 13) are given values which scale down their distance advantage, the corner regions (1, 6, 11, 16) are given a scale-up value, and the remainder are given a near neutral value. The same grouping occurs when $\lambda = 5$, however; for this solution there is less variation in their values, which reflects their tendency to return to neutral as $\lambda \to \infty$. This elimination of the locational effect arises because when $\lambda \to \infty$ all contacts tend to occur within each region.

The scalar values obtained for the observed population of Greater Manchester's regions reflect the effect of relative population conditional on location and the exponential decay parameter. When $\lambda = 0$, population size does not affect the neutral scalar values. However, for positive values of λ, the influence of the observed population can be ascertained by comparing the equivalent values of the observed and uniform scalars. For example, region 10 has a relatively small population in relation to its central location, such that the differences between the observed and uniform scalar values always indicate a decreased accessibility to the unevenly distributed population. Conversely, region 7 is more accessible in relation to the distribution of the observed population. Finally, the combination of a high-valued exponential decay parameter ($\lambda = 5$) and an uneven population produces extreme scalar values for the more sparsely populated corner regions to compensate for their increased separation from the rest of the system.

6.2 Time series simulations

6.2.1 *General behaviour* To understand how the various spatial representation systems influence the behaviour of the HD model, a series of simulations were conducted using the finite differencing methods described earlier. Some important general properties of the HD model can be illustrated by varying the starting values given to the epidemic populations. Figure 3 shows simulations obtained from the system with variable regional infectivity rates, S1, calibrated from the distribution of observed population (O) and with $\lambda = 1.3275$. For the sake of illustration, the epidemic is assumed to begin in region 4 with its equilibrium values of 7.99 carriers and 1.71 incubating infectives (see table 1). All other regions are given starting values of zero for their infective populations.

The 3 plots differ according to the starting values given to the susceptible populations, which were calculated from the relationship

$$x_{i,\,t\,=\,0} = x_i^{(0)} \pm a\left(y_i^{(0)} + z_i^{(0)}\right), \qquad \forall\, i \, . \tag{27}$$

Here, a denotes the units of the equilibrium infective populations that are either added to or subtracted from the equilibrium susceptible population in each region. The plots show the effect of setting a equal to 15, 0, and -15, successively.

An important property of the behaviour of the model not illustrated within the range of the plots is that, after their first major peak, the epidemic populations all exhibit a periodicity of 59 months, and the amplitude of subsequent peaks dampens with each cycle until equilibrium is reached. The period of 59 months is to be expected and is the same as that obtained from previous experiments (Thomas, 1986; 1988a) with this parameter set. Similarly, the dampening is typical of the behaviour of most deterministic models of disease (Bailey, 1975). These properties also arise if the systems S2 and S3 are employed (not illustrated) instead of S1. Another common feature is for all the regions (regions 3 and 4 are shown in figure 3) to reach the first major peak on each variable simultaneously. This effect can be delayed by choosing starting values which are excessively disproportionate from the distribution of the observed population. However, the symmetry of the spatial interaction components in the model ensures that, in the long run, the simulated regional epidemics will move into phase.

The carrier population of the starting region 4 falls after $t = 0$ because, with $y_{i, t = 0} = 0$, $\forall i \neq 4$, this region is a net 'exporter' of infections early on. This decline in the carrier population is passed on to near neighbours such as region 3, which experiences a minor carrier peak after a few months [see figures 3(a) and 3(c), for $a = 0$ and $a = -15$]. The incubating infective population experiences similar behaviour, with the exception that the removal of the starting population after an incubation period, k, of 3 months causes an early trough in the series for region 4. In each example the susceptible population grows steadily to a first major peak, at which point the infective populations are sufficiently large to induce a decline.

One effect of varying the starting values for the susceptible populations is to change the timing of the first major peak in each of the epidemic populations. For example, with starting values set above the equilibrium (that is, $a = 15$), the susceptibles peak early ($t = 7$), whereas starting

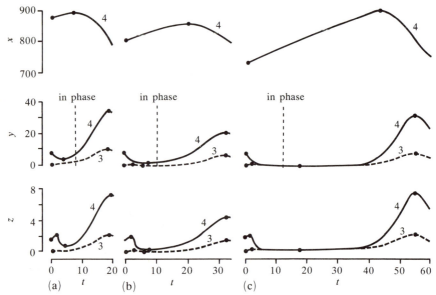

Figure 3. Plots of the simulated (S1) populations for alternative starting values of the number of susceptibles, $x_{i, t = 0}$, for the observed population (O) distribution, with $\lambda = 1.3275$: (a) $a = 15$; (b) $a = 0$; (c) $a = -15$. (See subsection 6.2.1 of text.)

values below the equilibrium $(a = -15)$ generate a late peak $(t = 43)$. In addition, the amplitudes of the epidemic populations increase at their first peak as the susceptible starting values move away from equilibrium $(a = 0)$. Such behaviour may be termed 'out of phase' because it depends on the degree of disequilibrium that is created by the choice of starting values.

An understanding of the outcomes of the spatial representation systems is facilitated by making the distinction between effects which occur when the regional series are out of phase with one another, and those which persist when these series are in phase. The relative change in the regional carrier populations is used to distinguish the two periods. Let $y_{i,t}/y_{i,t-1}$, $\forall i$, denote these changes; then the time when the series are taken to be in phase occurs when

$$\max\left(\frac{y_{i,t}}{y_{i,t-1}}\right) - \min\left(\frac{y_{i,t}}{y_{i,t-1}}\right) \leqslant 0.001 \ . \tag{28}$$

Although arbitrary, this definition is consistent and provides a basis for comparing different simulations. The positions of these times plotted on figure 3 show that the smaller the starting susceptible populations, the longer the carrier series take to become in phase.

6.2.2 *Out-of-phase effects* Figure 4 illustrates some of the major influences the 3 representation systems have on the simulated epidemic, for a distribution of both a uniform population (E) and the observed population (O). Notice the plots of the carrier population for the 3 systems diverge after $t = 0$ such that the first troughs are: for S1, at $y_{4,t=6.4} = 0.96$; for S2, at $y_{4,t=6.5} = 0.75$; and for S3, at $y_{4,t=6.8} = 0.80$. However, as the carrier populations move into phase $(t = 11.7)$, the plots for S2 and S3 merge. The plots for S1 (variable infectivity rates) stay separate from S2 and S3, and these differences will be examined subsequently as in-phase effects. The same broad pattern emerges for plots obtained from the distribution of the observed population (O), except the relatively large population of region 4 causes the troughs and peaks to appear earlier and with a higher amplitude; for example, for S1 the equivalent first trough for the observed population occurs at $y_{4,t=6.0} = 1.57$.

The plots for S2 and S3 differ from one another only as an out-of-phase effect. The nature of this difference can be demonstrated by comparing the first troughs already given for region 4 with those for the more inaccessible region 1. For a uniform population distribution these values are: for S2, $y_{1,t=8.7} = 0.99$; and for S3, $y_{1,t=7.9} = 0.90$. Because the carrier plots in both regions were obtained from the same starting value $(y_i = 7.99)$, the differences in timing are related to relative accessibility. It can be seen that the system S3 speeds up the progress of the epidemic in the relatively inaccessible region 1, but S3 delays the appearance of the first trough in region 4. However, the absolute differences between the

S2 and S3 series is so small that the choice between the systems for forecasting HD epidemics is likely to be immaterial.

A second out-of-phase effect is found by varying the value of the exponential decay parameter. Figure 5 and table 3 show how a selection of the regions, located at varying distances from the starting region 4, respond to the decay parameter. Figure 4 illustrates the outcomes for the system S1 where population is controlled by assuming a uniform distribution, E, over the regions. There is no decay effect when $\lambda = 0$,

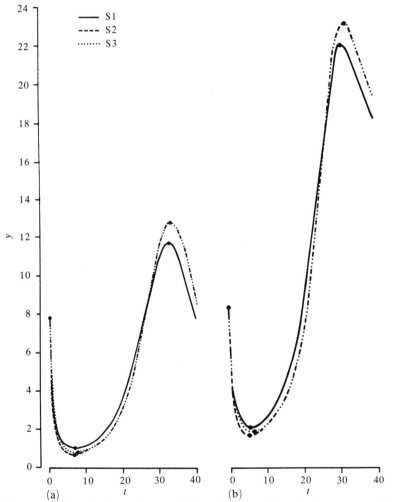

Figure 4. Plots of the carrier population of region 4 for the 3 representation systems (S1, S2, and S3) for (a) the distribution of a uniform population and (b) the distribution of the observed population, with $\lambda = 1.3275$ in each case.

and the starting region 4 moves into phase with the other regions ($\overline{4}$, see figure 5) at $t = 6$, soon after its first trough.

Let $\lambda = 5.0$, and the effects of distance decay become apparent. The out-of-phase period is now prolonged until $t = 63$ months and the regional epidemics respond according to their relative accessibility to the starting region. Table 3 shows that region 4 experiences a comparatively late first peak [at $t^{1P} = 34.7$ months] which arises because the chosen starting values induce an initial fall in the incidence of carriers. This effect also slows the growth of the carrier population in neighbouring regions, such as region 2, and combines with relative accessibility to region 4 to produce a sequence of first-peak times which does not correlate exactly with distance from the source of the epidemic, $d_{i,4}$. In addition, the amplitude of the regional carrier epidemics is also variable at their first peaks. With the exception of region 4, the amplitude of this peak increases in relation to the time of its occurrence. Thus the more inaccessible regions experience short, intense first epidemic waves in comparison with regions nearer to the source. The same correspondence between amplitude and time of the first peak does not apply to region 4, which exhibits the lowest amplitude of all the series, because its starting values induce a lag between the synchronisation of this region and all other regions. All these out-of-phase effects arise because higher values

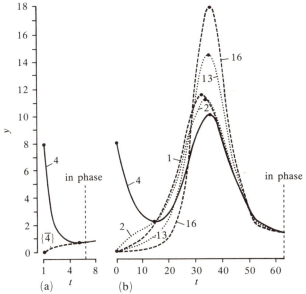

Figure 5. Plots of the carrier population, y, for selected regions, using the system S1 with a uniform population distribution for extreme values of the exponential decay parameter, λ: (a) $\lambda = 0$; (b) $\lambda = 5$.

of the exponential decay parameter increase the proportion of within-region contacts (Thomas, 1988a), such that regions respond more slowly to events elsewhere.

The results listed in table 3 show that the type of scaling system and population distribution also influence the timing and amplitude of the first peaks. However, it will be shown that these are persistent in-phase effects.

Table 3. Amplitude and time of the first peak of the carrier population under different scaling systems (S1 and S2) and population distributions (uniform, E, and observed, O) with $\lambda = 5.0$.

i	S1, E		S2, E		S1, O		S2, O		d_{i4}
	t^{1P}	y_i^{1P}	t^{1P}	y_i^{1P}	t^{1P}	y_i^{1P}	t^{1P}	y_i^{1P}	
4	34.7	10.0	35.0	10.2	34.5	18.3	34.7	19.5	0.4
2	33.6	11.1	33.7	11.3	33.7	8.7	33.7	9.5	1.0
1	32.5	11.6	32.6	11.8	32.3	9.3	32.7	10.3	1.4
13	34.6	14.6	34.8	14.8	33.3	34.1	34.0	35.6	1.4
16	35.0	18.3	35.2	18.5	33.3	2.4	34.1	2.6	2.8

Starting values ($t = 0$):
$y_4 = 8.0$ and $y_{i \neq 4} = 0.0$, $\forall i \neq 4$;
$z_4 = 1.7$ and $z_{i \neq 4} = 0.0$, $\forall i \neq 4$;
and
$x_i = x_i^{(0)}$, $\forall i$

Note: t^{1P} time of the first carrier peak; y_i^{1P} number of carriers at the first peak.

6.2.3 *In-phase effects* The most important effect occurs in relation to the behaviour of the simulated epidemic populations under the system S1 in comparison with the series obtained from S2 and S3. The effect concerns the time, t^P, and amplitude, y_i^P, of the peaks and troughs in the simulated series when identical starting values are given to each region in turn. Figure 6 illustrates the essential features of this locational variation where i' denotes the region given the positive starting values $y_{i'} = 8.0$ and $z_{i'} = 1.7$. For example, with a uniform population distribution, E, and S1 in operation, the first carrier peak occurs earlier and with a lower amplitude when $i' = 4$, than when $i' = 1$. This result reflects the higher accessibility of region 4 to the rest of the study area. However, under S2 (recall S3 gives identical results in the in-phase period) the carrier peaks occur at the same time, and with the same amplitude, irrespective of whether $i' = 4$ or $i' = 1$. The same pattern occurs when the distribution of the observed population (O) is introduced, although the time and amplitude are raised in proportion to the relatively higher population of region 4.

Table 4 is an extension of the graphical analysis and shows the outcome of locating the positive starting values in each of the 16 regions for S1 and S2 and for the distributions of the uniform and observed populations.

Applying S2 in conjunction with a uniform population distribution always leads us to a first peak at $t^{1P} = 33.3$ months, $\forall i$, with amplitude $y_i^{1P} = 1.29$, $\forall i$, irrespective of the starting region (i'). Replace S2 with S1, then the times and amplitudes of the first carrier peaks vary according to the locational accessibility of the source region.

Let S2 be used in conjunction with the observed population distribution, then the time of the first carrier peak remains constant at 33.3 but the amplitudes are now in proportion to the population, or average monthly incidence, of each region. Substitution of S1 for S2 creates a more complex outcome. First, the time of the first carrier peak varies according to the accessibility of the source region, which is indicated by the value of v_i, $\forall i$, for the observed population $(\lambda = 1.3275)$ as given in table 2. Second, the amplitude of the first carrier peak in each region will exceed the population proportional amplitude obtained from S2 whenever the time of the first peak for S1 is greater than the constant S2 time; and vice versa when the S1 time is less than the S2 time. In this way, lead and lag times induced by the relative accessibility of the source region cause variations in the amplitudes of the epidemic populations.

These results demonstrate the major consequence of the spatial representation systems. When variable infectivity rates (S1) are applied the epidemic peaks occur simultaneously in each region throughout the in-phase period; however, the time of these peaks will depend on the relative accessibility of the source region. Scaling the regional contact totals in line with a single set of study area rates (S2 and S3) again

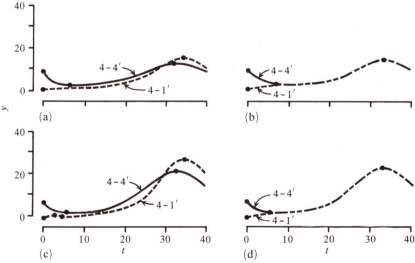

Figure 6. Plots of the carrier population in region 4 for simulations starting in region $i' = 1$ and $i' = 4$, with $\lambda = 1.3275$: (a) S1 with a uniform population; (b) S2 with a uniform population; (c) S1 with the observed population; (d) S2 with the observed population.

Table 4. Amplitude and time of the first peak of the carrier population under different scaling systems and population distributions.

i	i' with S1																i' with S2 and S3
	1'	2'	3'	4'	5'	6'	7'	8'	9'	10'	11'	12'	13'	14'	15'	16'	1'–16'

Uniform population distribution
Time of first carrier peak, t^{1P} (months):

i	1'	2'	3'	4'	5'	6'	7'	8'	9'	10'	11'	12'	13'	14'	15'	16'	1'–16'
1–16	33.9	33.3	33.3	32.8	33.3	33.9	32.8	33.3	33.3	32.8	33.9	33.3	32.8	33.3	33.3	33.9	33.3

Number of carriers at their first peak, y^{1P}:

i	1'	2'	3'	4'	5'	6'	7'	8'	9'	10'	11'	12'	13'	14'	15'	16'	1'–16'
1–16	14.0	12.9	12.9	11.9	12.9	14.0	11.9	12.9	12.9	11.9	14.0	12.9	11.9	12.9	12.9	14.0	12.9

Observed population distribution
Time of first carrier peak, t^{1P} (months):

i	1'	2'	3'	4'	5'	6'	7'	8'	9'	10'	11'	12'	13'	14'	15'	16'	1'–16'
1–16	34.8	33.8	34.2	32.9	33.7	34.7	32.6	33.5	34.6	33.0	35.8	34.2	32.7	33.8	33.9	35.1	33.3

Number of carriers at their first peak, y^{1P}:

i	1'	2'	3'	4'	5'	6'	7'	8'	9'	10'	11'	12'	13'	14'	15'	16'	1'–16'
1	12.8	11.5	12.1	10.2	11.5	12.8	9.8	11.2	12.7	10.5	14.3	12.2	10.0	11.6	11.8	13.5	10.6
2	12.4	11.1	11.7	9.8	11.0	12.3	9.4	10.8	12.2	10.1	13.8	11.7	9.6	11.1	11.3	13.0	10.4
3	8.1	7.3	7.6	6.4	7.2	8.1	6.2	7.1	7.8	6.6	9.0	7.6	6.3	7.3	7.4	8.5	6.8
4	27.4	24.5	25.7	21.5	24.2	27.1	20.7	23.7	26.7	22.1	30.2	25.6	21.0	24.4	24.8	28.4	22.9
5	14.4	12.9	13.6	11.4	12.6	14.2	10.9	12.4	14.1	11.6	15.9	13.5	11.1	12.8	13.1	14.9	12.1
6	5.8	5.2	5.4	4.6	5.1	5.6	4.3	4.9	5.6	4.7	6.4	5.4	4.4	5.1	5.2	6.0	4.8
7	35.6	31.9	33.5	28.0	31.4	35.1	26.8	30.6	34.8	28.7	39.2	33.3	27.2	31.6	32.2	36.8	29.9
8	21.1	19.0	20.0	16.7	18.7	20.8	15.9	18.1	20.7	17.1	23.3	19.8	16.2	18.7	19.2	21.9	17.8
9	5.8	5.2	5.4	4.5	5.1	5.7	4.4	5.0	5.6	4.6	6.3	5.4	4.4	5.1	5.2	6.0	4.8
10	22.6	20.3	21.2	17.8	20.0	22.4	17.1	19.5	22.0	18.1	24.9	21.0	17.2	20.1	20.4	23.4	19.0
11	1.4	1.3	1.4	1.1	1.3	1.4	1.1	1.2	1.4	1.2	1.6	1.3	1.1	1.3	1.3	1.5	1.2
12	12.5	11.2	11.8	9.9	11.1	12.4	9.5	10.8	12.2	10.0	13.7	11.5	9.5	11.1	11.2	12.9	10.5
13	37.1	33.3	34.9	39.2	32.7	36.6	27.9	31.9	36.1	29.8	40.8	34.5	28.2	32.8	22.4	38.2	31.2
14	11.6	10.4	10.9	9.1	10.2	11.4	8.7	9.9	11.3	9.3	12.7	10.8	8.8	10.2	10.4	11.9	9.7
15	14.9	13.4	14.0	11.8	13.2	14.7	11.3	12.9	14.5	12.0	16.4	13.8	11.3	13.2	13.4	15.3	12.6
16	2.4	2.2	2.3	1.9	2.1	2.4	1.8	2.1	2.3	1.9	2.6	2.2	1.8	2.1	2.2	2.5	2.0

Note: i' region infected at $t = 0$; $\lambda = 1.3275$. Starting values ($t = 0$): $y_{i'} = 8.0$ and $y_{i \neq i'} = 0.0$, $\forall i \neq i'$; $z_{i'} = 1.7$ and $z_{i \neq i'} = 0.0$, $\forall i \neq i'$; and $x_i = x_i^{(0)}$, $\forall i$.

causes simultaneous regional epidemic peaks, but now their timing is
constant irrespective of the accessibility of the source region. These
results all depend on the use of the same staring values for making the
comparison.

A related in-phase effect concerns the timing of the regional epidemic
peaks in relation to the value of the exponential decay parameter (figure 7).
Notice that with S2 or S3 in operation the time of the first epidemic
peak is a constant 33.3 months, irrespective of the value of λ. This result
again arises because the scaled contact totals make all the regions equally
accessible to one another. In contrast, regional infectivity rates (S1)
cause the timing to vary with the decay parameter such that relatively
inaccessible regions, like 1 and 2, experience delayed first carrier peaks.
The reverse is true for the relatively accessible regions, like region 4. The
size of the population in each region also influences this timing such
that regions with small populations in relation to their location experience
a further delay in the time of the first peak.

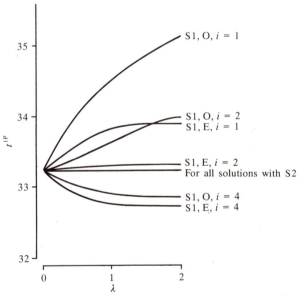

Figure 7. Plots of the time of the first carrier peak, t^{1P}, against the exponential
decay parameter, λ, for selected regions, using S1 and S2 for an observed (O) or
a uniform (E) population.

7 Discussion
It has been demonstrated that the alternative representations of the
infectivity rate(s) cause systematic variations to the simulated regional
epidemic time series. What remains to be established is the relative

significance of the effects induced by representation, and the performance of each system as a forecasting device.

The most important finding to emerge from the simulations is the relationship between the timing of the first epidemic peak and the location of the source region. This time is a constant with a single infectivity rate in operation (S2 and S3), but is variable when region-specific rates (S1) are applied. The choice between these two types of model behaviour ideally requires prior knowledge about contact patterns within the study area. For example, in large cities like Greater Manchester it might well be the case that higher peripheral contact propensities do cancel out regional accessibility differences. In such a circumstance S2 or S3 would be the appropriate model specification. Alternatively, region-specific rates would appear to provide the better option for predicting the path of a pandemic. It seems unlikely that the time of the first peak of an influenza pandemic beginning in Ulan Bator would be the same as one originating in Hong Kong. This speculation about the choice of representation system could be partially resolved by assessing how well stochastic versions of the models predicted the time of the first peak of an observed epidemic.

The simulations for HD in Greater Manchester showed that, in general, the time differences induced by varying the location of the source region were quite small. When λ was set to 1.3275, the difference between the maximum and minimum first peak times was 3.2 months [see table 4(b)], and occurred within a disease cycle of 59 months. However, the magnitude of this difference might well be sufficient to disrupt a disease control programme in which forecasts based on an inappropriate representation system are applied. Moreover, to establish the more general significance of the effect of the starting region, it would be instructive to calibrate the time differences for diseases with different periodicities and at a variety of spatial scales.

A further property of the Greater Manchester simulations was the strong tendency for the regional series to move quickly into phase such that, thereafter, each series was synchronised to the cycle obtained when the study area was represented as a single region: a result that indicates the capability of the spatial interaction components in the HD model for transforming out-of-phase starting values into a single cycle. This synchronisation is to be expected in a deterministic model where forecasts of the epidemic variables tend to their equilibrium values. However, it needs to be established whether stochastic versions of the model, which do not tend to equilibrium, exhibit the same behaviour. Similarly, although it has been shown how high values of the exponential decay parameter lengthen the out-of-phase period, this variation needs to be examined within a much more extensive study area than Greater Manchester.

The adoption of a stochastic modelling approach would also raise questions about the existence of the out-of-phase effects, which have been identified in relation to the configuration of starting values, the exponential decay parameter, and the choice of representation system. For example, these effects might be eliminated from the forecasts if the population of the study area were large enough to suggest the epidemic would not become extinct. Given this degree of endemnicity, then the stochastic forecasts could be fitted to the observed disease incidence by using methods I have described in an earlier paper (Thomas, 1988a). Initial forecasts for the regional series are obtained by using equilibrium starting values. These series are then aggregated and matched to the series of disease incidence in the study area in accordance with their cross-correlation function. In this way the stochastic model is fitted directly to the observed 'in-phase' disease cycle. Alternatively, for applications where extinction is observed, good estimates of all the starting values will be required, and the deterministic simulation of the out-of-phase effects will be a necessary precursor to understanding the variances of the stochastic forecasts.

The comments so far all refer to the internal functioning of the models. However, this space–time modelling system can be extended in line with the existing body of spatial interaction theory (Wilson and Bennett, 1985). For example, an estimate of the total travel distance, D, undertaken while making contacts within the study area in a unit of time, would enable the constraint

$$\sum_{i,j}^{m} C_{ij}^{(0)} d_{ij} = D \, , \tag{29}$$

to apply in conjunction the equilibrium regional contact totals defined by equation (14). These constraints can be satisfied by the application of entropy-maximising or information-minimising principles to obtain a unique value of λ in equation (15), and a set of scalars, A_i, $\forall i$, which are consistent with observed travel behaviour in the study area.

Spatial interaction models with similar functional forms can be derived from a plethora of economic and statistical assumptions as demonstrated by Bröker's (1989) recent synthesis. This variety suggests that the possibilities for their representation in multiregion disease models extends far beyond the methods that have been tested here. The task will be to identify parsimonious forms which are the most appropriate for different diseases and spatial scales. It might also be the case that the temporal mechanisms contained in a disease model have counterparts in economic systems; for example, the spread of an innovation has many parallels with the progress of an epidemic.

Acknowledgements. Thanks are due to Graham Bowden for preparing the diagrams.

References

Bailey N J T, 1975 *The Mathematical Theory of Infectious Diseases* (Charles Griffin, London)

Baroyan O V, Rvachev L A, 1967, "Deterministic epidemic models for a territory with a transport network" *Kibernetika* **3** 67–74

Bartlett M S, 1960 *Stochastic Population Models in Ecology and Epidemiology* (Methuen, Andover, Hants)

Bröker J, 1989, "Partial equilibrium theory of interregional trade and the gravity model" *Papers of the Regional Science Association* **66** 7–18

Cliff A D, Haggett P, Ord J K, 1986 *Spatial Aspects of Influenza Epidemics* (Pion, London)

Cliff A D, Haggett P, Ord J K, Versey G R, 1981 *Spatial Diffusion: An Historical Geography of Epidemics in an Island Community* (Cambridge University Press, Cambridge)

Greenberg R S, Grufferman S, Cole P, 1983, "An evaluation of space–time clustering in Hodgkin's Disease" *Journal of Chronic Disease* **36** 257–262

Grufferman S, Delzell E, 1984, "Epidemiology of Hodgkin's Disease" *Epidemiology Review* **6** 76–106

MacMahon B, 1966, "Epidemiology of Hodgkin's Disease" *Cancer Research* **26** 1189–1200

Mangoud A, Hillier V, Leck I, Thomas R W, 1985, "Space–time interaction in Hodgkin's Disease in Greater Manchester" *Journal of Epidemiology and Community Health* **39** 58–62

Masser I, Brown P J B, 1977, "Spatial representation and spatial interaction" *Papers of the Regional Science Association* **38** 71–92

Murray G D, Cliff A D, 1977, "A stochastic model for measles epidemics in a multi-regin setting" *Transactions of the Institute of British Geographers: New Series* **2** 158–174

Rvachev L A, Longini I M, 1985, "A mathematical model for the global spread of influenza" *Mathematical Biosciences* **75** 3–22

Smith P G, Pike M C, 1976, "Current epidemiological evidence for transmission of Hodgkin's Disease" *Cancer Research* **36** 660–662

Thomas R W, 1986, "A single-region carrier model for the simulation of Hodgkin's Disease applied to its incidence in Greater Manchester, 1962–1976" *Environment and Planning A* **18** 929–948

Thomas R W, 1988a, "Stochastic carrier models for the simulation of Hodgkin's Disease in a system of regions" *Environment and Planning A* **20** 1575–1601

Thomas R W, 1988b, "Carrier models for the simulation of Hodgkin's Disease: a review with some extensions" *Social Science and Medicine* **26** 131–140

Thomas R W, 1990, "Some spatial representation problems in disease modelling" *Geographical Analysis* **22**

Vianna N J, 1975 *Lymphoreticular Malignancies* (Medical and Technical Publishing, Lancaster)

Wilson A G, Bennett R J, 1985 *Mathematical Methods in Human Geography and Planning* (John Wiley, Chichester, Sussex)

Part 3

The AIDS Pandemic

Acquired Immunodeficiency Syndrome (AIDS): The Global Spread of Human Immunodeficiency Virus Type 2 (HIV-2)

M R SMALLMAN-RAYNOR, A D CLIFF
University of Cambridge

1 Introduction

1.1 Background

The year 1984 marked an important advance in our understanding of Acquired Immunodeficiency Syndrome or AIDS. The disease had first been recognised clinically in 1979 in a patient in a New York hospital who died after a long and mysterious sickness characterised by repeated attacks of chance infections which are usually easily repelled by the body. Cross-checks with other United States hospitals revealed not only an alarming number of similar cases, but also a steep rise in hospital admissions of patients suffering from illness which pointed to collapse of the immune system. Because of this the new disease received its name, acquired immunodeficiency syndrome, and over the decade since 1979 it has reached global pandemic proportions.

The causative agent of AIDS was at first a mystery. In 1984, however, scientists in France and America were reporting the isolation of a virus from AIDS patients. Within two years this complex virus, later to be termed human immunodeficiency virus type 1 (HIV-1), was recognised as the causative agent underlying the emergence of the global AIDS pandemic, and it appeared initially to be the sole such agent.

In 1986, just as a picture of the global epidemiology of AIDS and associated HIV-1 infection was emerging, French scientists were observing West African patients with the now all-too-familiar illnesses suggestive of AIDS. A few months later, these scientists announced the isolation of a related but genetically distinct 'second' AIDS virus, human immuno-deficiency virus type 2 (HIV-2), from the same patients. Thus within two years of AIDS being recognised as a viral disease of pandemic proportions, a new area of AIDS research had been born.

There are three main transmission corridors by which HIV, covering both strains of the virus, is passed from person to person, although there is some evidence of between-strain variability in the efficiency of transmission (appendix 1). The first corridor is through sexual contact with an infected person. Most bodily fluids act as a reservoir for the virus so that both homosexual and heterosexual relations with an HIV carrier can result in spread. The second corridor is through contact with contaminated blood or blood products. Given the screening of blood in the hospital services of western nations, the most common way that infected blood transfer occurs in these countries is via the habit of sharing syringes among intravenous drugs abusers (IVDAs), although the use of untreated blood products remains a problem in the developing world. The third corridor, emerging as the major route after heterosexual transmission in some African and Caribbean countries, is perinatal infection of infants by an infected mother.

The reproductive mechanism of HIV in the human body kills certain of the white blood cells known as T4 lymphocytes which form a crucial part of the human immune system. This lays the body open to a wide range of chance infections, as well as to specific types of autoimmune and neurological disorders and to several types of malignancy including the diagnostic Kaposi's sarcoma.

Uncertainty surrounds the relative pathogenic potential (the disease-causing capability) of HIV-1 and HIV-2. Both strains appear to have extraordinarily long incubation periods. However, provided other causes of death do not prematurely intervene, it is believed in the present state of medical knowledge that mortality from HIV disease is certain for those infected with HIV-1. In contrast, reports of the pathogenic capability of HIV-2 are conflicting. This uncertain status of HIV-2 infection has important implications for the international response to the second strain of the AIDS virus, and the debate surrounding its pathogenicity is outlined in appendix 1.

In the years following the first reports of AIDS and the isolation of HIV-1, the growth of the epidemic has been immense. By 30 June 1989, some 167 000 AIDS cases associated with HIV-1 had been reported to the World Health Organization (WHO, 1989), from 149 countries around the world; however, WHO estimates that, because of underreporting, the true number of cases is closer to 350 000 (Mann, personal communication, 1989)[1] and that a further 5 to 10 million people are infected with HIV-1. A clear picture of the global HIV-1 epidemic is now emerging.

In contrast, the global HIV-2 epidemic appears still to be in its infancy. By January 1988, when over 75 000 cases of AIDS associated with HIV-1 AIDS had been reported to WHO (WHO, 1988), only 44 cases of AIDS associated with HIV-2 had been described in the literature, with a further 639 documented infections (Horsburgh and Holmberg, 1988). By the end of June 1989, only 0.5% of the world's reported AIDS cases had been recorded from areas of known endemic HIV-2 infection and many of these were attributable to HIV-1. Yet it is already clear that, as with HIV-1, the HIV-2 epidemic is far more widespread than published figures indicate. For example, de la Cruz et al (1989) estimate that there are 15 000–20 000 HIV-2 infections in Mozambique

[1] Dr J Mann can be contacted at WHO Global Programme on AIDS, World Health Organization, Geneva.

alone, a country only recently recognised as displaying endemic HIV-2 infection.

1.2 Rationale and layout of paper

This paper is designed to introduce geographers to a subfield of AIDS research that may have a future major bearing on our understanding of the epidemiology of the disease. Given the apparently limited geographical extent and uncertain pathogenic significance of the current HIV-2 epidemic, it may seem surprising to focus attention on this AIDS virus. Yet, there are good reasons for doing so. First, it is already apparent that HIV-2 displays a geography clearly distinct from HIV-1 and, at the time of writing, no attempt has been made to review its known geography. Second, HIV-2 has been hypothesised as a key link in the emergence of HIV-1 (Essex and Kanki, 1988) and this may have a significant impact upon our understanding of the emergence of the global AIDS pandemic. Third, in the late 1970s and early 1980s the global diffusion of HIV-1 caught the world by surprise, and attempts to reconstruct the corridors of spread of this virus are limited by the quality of early epidemiological data (see Smallman-Raynor and Cliff, 1990a; 1990b). HIV-2, in contrast, offers a unique possibility for the reconstruction of the diffusion of a virus in a nascent pandemic.

In the first section of this paper, we outline the completeness of the global picture of HIV-2 infection and associated AIDS occurrence as discussed in the medical literature. In subsequent sections, we examine the evidence regarding the likely geographical origins of HIV-2; we outline the known spatial occurrence and global epidemiology of HIV-2 infection and contrast it with that of HIV-1; we reconstruct the major diffusion poles and corridors of spread of an embryonic pandemic; and we present a general time-dependent spread model of HIV-2 from the hypothesised hearth of the virus, based upon our reconstruction of the diffusion corridors. In the conclusion to the paper, we outline a number of research questions that may be profitably pursued by geographers involved in AIDS research.

2 AIDS and HIV-2 infection: global literature coverage

2.1 *Literature growth*

The literature relating to AIDS has grown explosively over the last 8 years. With well over 10 000 publications cited in the western world's major medical publication index, the United States National Library of Medicine's *Cumulated Index Medicus*, literature growth has outstripped that relating to any other disease. [See Smallman-Raynor and Cliff (1990a) for an examination of trends.]

Comparison of the growth of literature relating to HIV-2 with that for all AIDS literature can be made by analysis of citations in a publication of the Bureau of Hygiene and Tropical Disease, *AIDS and Retroviruses*

Update/Current AIDS Literature[2]. Trends are shown in figure 1. Research on HIV-2 is clearly still in its infancy. Despite rapid growth over a 30-month period between 1987 and 1989, little over 1% of all AIDS literature cited refers to HIV-2 and less than 0.8% of all cited literature is relevant to the epidemiology or occurrence of this virus.

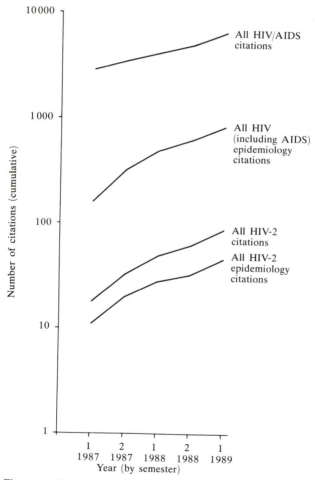

Figure 1. Growth in all AIDS literature compared with literature relating to HIV-2, 1987–89 (log scale). Sources: BHTD, 1986–87; CS/BHTD, 1988–89.

[2] *AIDS and Retroviruses Update/Current AIDS Literature* is one of the world's leading AIDS abstracting publications. Initiated as *AIDS and Retroviruses Update* in 1986 and renamed *Current AIDS Literature* in 1988, over 1400 journals published globally are surveyed in the publication.

2.2 Global literature coverage

A restricted literature on HIV-2 translates into limited knowledge of the global distribution of the virus. Figure 2 shows the growth of literature referring to the epidemiology of HIV-1 and HIV-2 by continent. Over a 30-month period to the end of June 1989 the ratio of HIV-1 to HIV-2 literature stood at 8 : 1 for Europe, 6 : 1 for Africa, and 47 : 1 for the Americas. Over 55% of all HIV-2 epidemiological literature has focused on Europe, with less than 13% referring to the Americas, Asia, and Oceania.

A more complete global coverage emerges if analysis is extended to include conference presentations and newsletter reports. Figure 3 shows a total of 60 countries drawn from over 100 sources for which information on the epidemiology of HIV-2 infection was available by 30 June 1989. Virtually the whole of sub-Saharan Africa, North America, and Western Europe is represented, although reports from elsewhere in the world are sporadic.

Nevertheless, despite the currently still-fragmented nature of this global picture, a distinct geography of HIV-2 infection is beginning to emerge, and it is to this which we now turn.

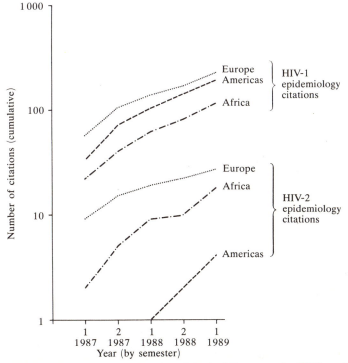

Figure 2. Growth in AIDS epidemiological literature by HIV strain and world region, 1987–89 (log scale). Sources: BHTD, 1986–87; CS/BHTD, 1988–89.

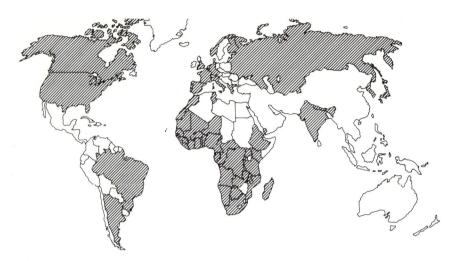

Figure 3. Countries (cross-shaded) for which HIV-2 screening has been reported. Sources: see appendix 4, subsection A4.1.

3 The age and geographical origins of HIV-2

3.1 Origins of HIV-2

From the time of the first reports of AIDS in US homosexuals in 1981 (Gottlieb et al, 1981; Hymes et al, 1981; Masur et al, 1981; Siegal et al, 1981) and the first reports of the isolation of HIV (Barré-Sinoussi et al, 1983; Gallo et al, 1984; Levy et al, 1984; Vilmer et al, 1984), the origins of the virus and the disease have been of intense interest, speculation, and contention. A number of hypotheses have been proposed regarding the likely origins of HIV, and these are discussed in appendix 2. In this section we focus upon the implications for the hearth of HIV-2 should the presently most widely-held view that HIV is a mutation of viruses endemic in certain species of wild African monkey be correct.

A search for the hearth of HIV-2 is made simpler than that for HIV-1 given the apparently restricted global spread of the virus. Whereas most virological and epidemiological evidence points to a Central African hearth for HIV-1 (for an overview, see Smallman-Raynor and Cliff, 1990a; 1990b), HIV-2 was first isolated in 1986 from AIDS patients originating from the former Portuguese West African colonies of Cape Verde and Guinea-Bissau (Clavel et al, 1986), with early serological evidence suggesting that HIV-2 was uniquely endemic to this part of the continent (Clavel, 1987). Subsequent serological analysis has confirmed the endemic nature of HIV-2 infection in West Africa, with the detection of a major subpole of infection in the former Portuguese South Central African colonies of Angola and Mozambique (see subsection 5.1 below).

In recent times a number of simian immunodeficiency viruses (SIVs) have been detected and isolated in wild African species of monkey.

As discussed in appendix 2, the strongest evidence for the origin of
HIV-2 comes from the recent detection in the *wild* of an SIV, SIVman,
first isolated in 1986 from *captive* African sooty mangabeys (*Cercocebus
atys*) (see Hirsch et al, 1989; Li et al, 1989; Murphey-Corb et al, 1986).
SIVman and HIV-2 share such an extrordinarily close genetic homology
that Hirsch et al (1989) and Li et al (1989) argue forcefully that the
sooty mangabey is the direct ancestor host of HIV-2.

The geographical implications of this hypothesis are illustrated in
figure 4 in which the major areas of known HIV-2 endemic infection are
compared with the natural range of the sooty mangabey. The monkey's
natural range coincides with the area of West Africa displaying the
highest rates of HIV-2 infection, including southern Senegal, Guinea-
Bissau, and Ivory Coast. Indeed, Clavel (1987) tentatively suggests that
Guinea-Bissau may be the hearth of HIV-2 because of the extent of the
penetration of the virus into the general human population of this country.
The high degree of genetic homology shared by HIV-2 and SIVman, and
the coincidence of a major area of endemic HIV-2 infection with the
natural range of the sooty mangabey, suggests that West Africa is the
hearth of HIV-2 and that the sooty mangabey is the ancestor host.

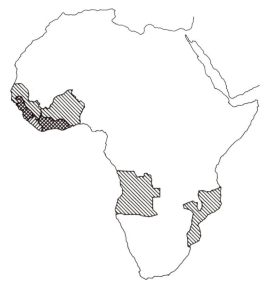

▨ Known natural range of sooty mangabey (*Cercocebus atys*) (see Wolfheim, 1983)
▧ Known areas of endemic HIV-2 infection (various sources)
▦ Both categories

Figure 4. The hearth of HIV-2, with known areas of endemic HIV-2 infection in
Africa and the natural range of the sooty mangabey (*Cercocebus atys*). Sources:
de la Cruz et al, 1989; Fleming, 1988; Matos-Almeida et al, 1989; Romieu
et al, 1989; Woflheim, 1983.

3.2 The age of HIV-2

Like its sister virus, HIV-1, the age of HIV-2 remains an area of speculation. Analysis of the likely sources and dates of infection of early European HIV-2 seropositives implies that the virus was circulating in West and South Central Africa in the 1960s (Ancelle et al, 1987; Bryceson et al, 1988; Saimot et al, 1987). This view is supported by retrospective serological analysis (Kawamura et al, 1989) and SIVman is also known to have been present in colonies of captive sooty mangabeys in the United States of America in the same decade (Hirsch et al, 1989). Although this may be taken as an indication of a minimum emergence date, phylogenetic histories of retroviruses are variable in their estimation of time of emergence, ranging between 1710 and 1950 AD, and with an indication that HIV-2 may be an older virus than HIV-1 (Smith et al, 1988; Yokoyama et al, 1988).

4 The spatial occurrence of HIV-2

4.1 Global overview

Detail relating to the occurrence of HIV-2 infection is available for 60 countries, or one-third of the countries officially reporting AIDS cases to the World Health Organization. In figure 5(a), those countries from which unique HIV-2 infection[3] has been documented are shown. Most of West and South Central Africa, Western Europe, North America, the USSR, and Brazil have reported the existence of HIV-2 infection within their borders. However, only about 220 of the approximately 2000 HIV-2 infections detailed in 75 reports occur outside the 2 principal regions of endemic infection of West Africa and Angola/Mozambique. A further 5 countries have reported only 'dual' HIV-1/HIV-2 infection [figure 5(b)].

This global pattern of HIV-2 occurrence and endemicity contrasts markedly with that of HIV-1; HIV-1 infection heartlands include North and South America, the Caribbean, Western Europe, and Central Africa. In the USA and Western Europe alone there are estimated to be between 1 million and 2 million HIV-1 infections, and WHO forecasts 250 000 HIV-1 related deaths by the mid-1990s in a 'typical' Central African country with a population of 20 million (CDC, 1989; Chin and Mann, 1989).

[3] 'Unique HIV-2 infection' refers to infection in the absence of evidence of HIV-1. 'Apparent dual HIV-1/HIV-2 infection' may arise because of antigenic cross-reactivity in the application of serological testing procedures (appendix 1). All HIV-2 infections referred to subsequently are unique HIV-2 infections, unless stated otherwise.

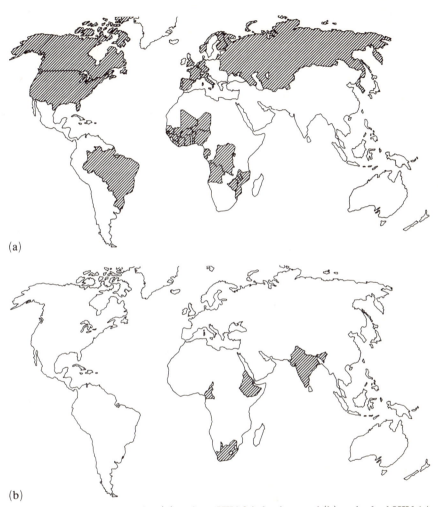

Figure 5. Countries reporting (a) unique HIV-2 infection, and (b) only dual HIV-1/ HIV-2 infection within their borders. Sources: see appendix 4, subsection A4.2.

5 The spatial occurrence of HIV-2 in Africa

5.1 HIV infection and AIDS: continental overview

The heartlands of HIV-1 and HIV-2 infection in Africa are geographically distinct (figure 6). From the time of the pioneering studies in Zaire (Piot et al, 1984) and Rwanda (Van de Perre et al, 1984) serological analysis has confirmed Central Africa as being a primary pole of HIV-1 infection and associated AIDS. Figure 6 shows a delimitation of this heartland based upon serological surveys. The heartland reaches from the Central African Republic in the north to Zambia and Malawi in the south, and from Kenya/Tanzania in the east to Congo in the west.

Some 3 years after the first isolations of HIV-2 in AIDS patients
from the former Portuguese West African colonies of Guinea-Bissau and
Cape Verde (Clavel et al, 1986), the picture of infection with this second
virus is still far from complete. However, there appear to be 2 distinct,
but historically linked, regions of endemic infection: the hypothesised
hearth of the virus in West Africa and the 2 former Portuguese colonies
of Angola and Mozambique in southern Central Africa (figure 6).

Serological surveys for HIV-2 in Central Africa suggest that infection
with the virus is very rare in this part of the continent (see, for example,
Kanki et al, 1987). HIV-1 has recently penetrated some West African
states (table A1, appendix 3), probably through importation from Europe
(see subsection 5.2 below). In some West African cohorts, for example
in the Ivory Coast, HIV-1 penetration has reached parity with HIV-2
(Ouattara et al, 1989), and in Ghana HIV-1 penetration exceeds that of
HIV-2 (Fleming, 1988). In yet others, such as Senegal, the principal virus
appears to be HIV-2 (Kanki et al, 1989).[4]

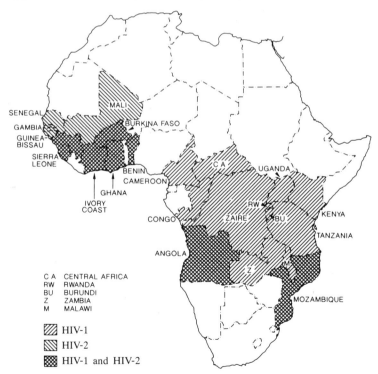

Figure 6. Location of HIV-1 and HIV-2 infection heartlands in Africa. Sources:
principally from de la Cruz et al, 1989; Fleming, 1988; Matos-Almeida et al,
1989; Romieu et al, 1989.

[4] Detail on epidemiological aspects of HIV-2 in African countries appears in
appendix 3.

The continental variation in the penetration of HIV-1 and HIV-2, coupled with the possibly limited pathogenic potential of the second AIDS virus, parallels a distinct geography in the continental occurrence of AIDS. By the end of June 1989, 86% of the 30 064 African AIDS cases had been reported from the Central African heartland for HIV-1. Conversely, only 6.6% of cases had been reported from countries displaying endemic HIV-2 infection, and many of these may be attributed to HIV-1 infection (WHO, 1989). In Ivory Coast, for example, the prevalences of HIV-1 and HIV-2 infection in the general population are approximately equal, although studies of hospitalised AIDS cases have shown almost 90% to be associated with HIV-1 (Gody et al, 1988). Similarly, two-thirds of Mozambique's 72 AIDS cases reported to May 1989 have been associated with HIV-1 infection, despite an estimated level of HIV-2 infections twice that of HIV-1 in the major urban centres of the country (16 700 versus 9 700; see de la Cruz et al, 1989). Nevertheless, in countries such as Gambia, AIDS cases associated with HIV-2 have outstripped those due to HIV-1 (figure 7) such that, by March 1989, the ratio of AIDS cases associated with HIV-2 to those associated with HIV-1 stood at 3.5 : 1 (Oelman et al, 1989).

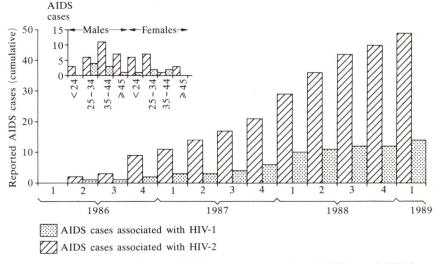

Figure 7. Cumulative number of AIDS cases associated with HIV-1 and HIV-2 reported quarterly in the Gambia, January 1986 to March 1989. Source: drawn from Oelman et al, 1989.

5.2 The diffusion of HIV-2 infection in Africa
Although there is strong evidence to support the hypothesis that HIV-1 was introduced into West African nations, probably directly from Europe rather than from Central Africa, in the mid-1980s (for example, see Fultz et al, 1988; Konotey-Ahulu, 1989; Mabey et al, 1988; Ouattara

et al, 1986), HIV-2 infection is known to have been circulating in Senegal
and Guinea-Bissau in the 1970s (Fultz et al, 1988; M'Boup et al, 1989).
In many countries of the region which now display endemic HIV-2
infection, there is no evidence of AIDS/HIV infection prior to 1985–86.
This suggests only recent spread of HIV into these countries (Gody et al,
1988; Konotey-Ahulu, 1989; Mabey et al, 1988; Neequaye et al, 1986).

A reconstruction of the likely diffusion poles and corridors of spread
of HIV-2 on the continent appears in figure 8. For many countries
reporting the existence of HIV-2 infection within their borders, appropriate
data on infection sources are not available. However, from the information
that is available, the diffusion of HIV-2 in Africa appears to have differed
markedly from that of HIV-1. The spread of HIV-1 has focused upon a
Central African diffusion pole (Smallman-Raynor and Cliff, 1990b).
HIV-2, in contrast, appears to have followed a 2-way drift, eastwards
and southwards, from an infection pole pivoted upon Guinea-Bissau and
Senegal (see figure 6 for locations).

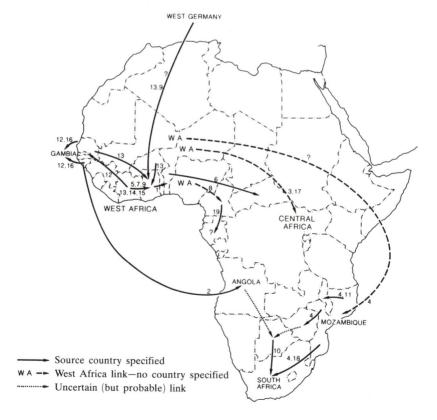

Figure 8. The diffusion of HIV-2 within Africa. Sources: see numbered references
in appendix 4, subsection A4.3.

In West Africa, eastward drift from Guinea-Bissau/Senegal has occurred into other countries of endemic HIV-2 infection: Gambia, Ivory Coast, Ghana, Benin, and Burkina Faso. Additional, if still limited, eastward spread from West Africa into Niger, Nigeria, and the Northwest Central African states of Cameroon, Gabon, and Central African Republic is indicated by sporadic reports of infection linked to West Africa.

International prostitution as the central vector for HIV-2 diffusion in West Africa is implicated in reports from Gambia (Pepin et al, 1989), Benin (Bigot et al, 1987), Ivory Coast (Denis et al, 1987), and Ghana (Ishikawa et al, 1988; Konotey-Ahulu, 1989; Neequaye et al, 1988). In Ghana, for example, the epidemiological characteristics of the HIV epidemic strongly support this hypothesis. Ishikawa et al (1988) report on the isolation of HIV-2 from a Ghanaian female prostitute whose only work had been conducted in Abidjan (Ivory Coast), and to the end of 1987 there were a total of 276 known HIV infections in the country. Of these, almost 200 were female prostitutes who had returned with disease from the Ivory Coast, giving an extraordinary male : female sex ratio for known infections of 1 : 7.6 (Neequaye et al, 1988).

The spread of HIV-2 southwards into the former Portuguese colonies of Angola and Mozambique in South Central Africa appears to have occurred directly from the West African hearth of HIV-2, carried there by Portuguese. The centrality of the Portuguese link is supported by the fact that the earliest reported HIV-2 infection in Angola was in a Portuguese male who had previously been resident in the former Portuguese colony of Guinea-Bissau (Böttiger et al, 1988). There is also evidence that the historically strong connections between Portugal and Mozambique have been central to the diffusion of HIV-2 from West Africa to this part of the continent (de la Cruz, personal communiction[5]). Subsequently, these subpoles of HIV-2 infection appear to have acted as diffusion poles in the spread of the virus northwards into Malawi and southwards into Southern Africa (de la Cruz, personal communication, see footnote 5; Lyons et al, 1988b; 1989).

6 The spatial occurrence of HIV-2 in Europe
6.1 HIV infection and AIDS: continental overview
Europe is a global heartland of HIV-1 infection. By the end of June 1989, over 22 000 AIDS cases associated with HIV-1 had been reported to WHO, with a minimum estimate in 1987 of 0.5 million HIV-1 infections in the continent (Chin and Mann, 1989). In contrast, the European HIV-2 epidemic appears still to be in its infancy. However, extensive serological surveys for the infection have not been conducted for ethical and economic reasons, coupled with uncertainties surrounding the disease-causing potential of the virus. Exceptions are Portugal and France.

[5] Dr F de La Cruz may be contacted at the Immunology Laboratory, Instituto Nacional de Saude, Maputo, Mozambique.

Only 5 European countries had reported the existence of HIV-2 within their borders by the end of January 1988. Together, 32 cases of HIV-2 infection, including 6 AIDS cases and 1 case of AIDS-related complex (ARC) had been reported in Europe by this date (Horsburgh and Holmberg, 1988; Kingman, 1987; Vittecoq et al, 1987). European HIV-2 infections noted in the literature to June 1989, based upon the sources for figure 5(a), are listed in appendix 3. The number of specified unique infections had grown to over 200 (including possible repeat reports) by this date, established from over 140 000 conducted tests in 12 countries (table A3, appendix 3). Portugal alone has reported 19 cases of AIDS associated with HIV-2 (Ayres et al, 1989). A further 160 cases of 'dual' HIV-1/HIV-2 infection had been recorded, 132 of them from Italy (table A4, appendix 3). Most of these dual infections are, however, believed to be attributable to the cross-reactivity problem (appendix 1).

Undoubtedly the extent of HIV-2 infection in Europe is far more extensive than these figures would suggest, but the early reported cases of infection are central to the reconstruction of the major diffusion poles and corridors of spread of a nascent epidemic.

6.2 Diffusion of HIV-2 in Europe

A reconstruction of the diffusion of HIV-2 into Europe, based upon a subset of the 205 unique HIV-2 infectious listed in table A3 (appendix 3), is shown in figure 9. Sufficient epidemiological information is available for 155 cases to determine a continent of infection, of which 129 are believed to have been imported into Europe. An epidemiological breakdown of 81 of these externally linked infections is shown in table 1. The critical role of West Africa, the hypothesised hearth of the virus, as a diffusion pole in the spread of HIV-2 into Europe is clear, with a subpole focused upon Angola/Mozambique. All imported cases are linked to Africa; over 90% are linked to West Africa, and nearly 72% of the infections are among West Africans in Europe.

Portugal is the only European country with an established HIV-2 epidemic. Almost 10% of 199 reported AIDS cases in that country to the end of 1988 were attributed to HIV-2 infection, and prevalence

Table 1. Believed region of infection and nationality for 81 cases of unique HIV-2 infection in Europe. Sources: see table A3, appendix 3.

Source region	Nationality		Total
	Europeans	Africans	
West Africa	15	58	73
Angola/Mozambique	4	1	5
Central Africa	1	2	3

studies have indicated that the virus has entered all risk groups within the country (table 2). As with the spread of HIV-2 in Africa, Portugal has acted as a central cog in the diffusion of the virus into the European continent. More than 55% of unique HIV-2 infections for which a likely source country is stated and which are listed in table A3 are linked to the former Portuguese colonies of Guinea-Bissau, Cape Verde, Mozambique, and Angola. A total of 17 of the 26 externally linked HIV-2 infections for which European nationality is specified have occurred in Portuguese natives. Indeed, the earliest detected HIV-2 infections in Europe were Portuguese natives having had direct contact with former Portuguese colonies in Africa (Ancelle et al, 1987; Bryceson et al, 1988; Saimot et al, 1987), and there is evidence that Portugal has acted as a major stepping stone for the international HIV-2 diffusion within Europe (Dufoort et al, 1988; Simon et al, 1989b).

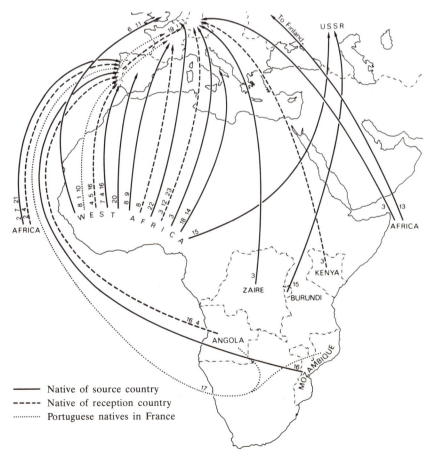

Figure 9. The diffusion of HIV-2 into Europe. Sources: see numbered references in appendix 4, subsection A4.4.

Table 2. Results of serological screening for HIV-1 and HIV-2 infection, conducted in Portugal.

Group	Date	Location	Number screened	Number HIV positive	
				HIV-1	HIV-2
Attenders of STD clinics[a]:					
Female prostitutes	1986–88	Lisbon	302		6 (2.0%)
Male homosexuals or bisexuals	1986–88	Lisbon	68		0 (0.0%)
Male heterosexuals	1986–88	Lisbon	557		1 (0.2%)
Blood donor units[b]	1985–87	Lisbon	43 533	12 (0.028%)	
Blood donor units[b]	1987	Lisbon	8196		3 (0.03%)
National screening programme[c]:					
Homosexuals	to Dec. 1988	All	210	60 (28.6%)	2 (1.0%)
Intravenous drug abusers	to Dec. 1988	All	1239	113 (9.1%)	4 (0.3%)
Prostitutes	to Dec. 1988	All	214	3 (1.4%)	2 (0.9%)
Heterosexuals	to Dec. 1988	All	75	12 (16.0%)	16 (21.3%)
Pregnants	to Dec. 1988	All	572	3 (0.5%)	4 (0.7%)

Note: STD sexually transmitted disease, Dec. December.
[a] Cardoso et al, 1989.
[b] Ayres et al, 1989.
[c] Torres Pereira and Louro Rodrigues, 1988.

If West and South Central Africa have acted as major diffusion poles for HIV-2 into Europe, there is also evidence, albeit still limited, of the spread of infection within the European continent (internal infection). Only 26 infections for which there is sufficient epidemiological information and which are listed in table A3 may be attributed to internal infection and, in many of these cases, indirect African contact is either known or cannot be ruled out. In addition to Portugal, likely internal infections have also been reported from Italy, the USSR, and Belgium from all groups at risk for HIV-1 infection. In France, there have been reports of HIV-2 infection transmitted via whole blood (Dufoort et al, 1988; Rouzioux et al, 1989) and blood products (Simon et al, 1989b; Tricoire et al, 1989), with the possibility that HIV-2 was circulating among the native homosexual population as early as 1984–85 (Brücker et al, 1987; Rey et al, 1987). It is also evident that international prostitution is playing a part in the importation and diffusion of the virus within European populations (Vittecoq et al, 1987).

The diffusion poles in the development of the nascent European HIV-2 epidemic already appear to be substantially different from those for HIV-1. Reconstructions of diffusion poles and corridors of spread of HIV-1 into Europe in the early stages of the AIDS pandemic have implicated the USA as the principal diffusion pole, with Central Africa and Haiti as subpoles (Smallman-Raynor and Cliff, 1990a; 1990b).

7 The spatial occurrence of HIV-2 in the Americas and Asia
7.1 HIV-2 in the Americas
Transvestite homosexual male prostitutes resident in Sao Paulo, Brazil, represent the earliest reported detections of unique HIV-2 infection in the Americas (Veronesi et al, 1987). Some 2 years after this first report, results of HIV-2 screening were published for just 5 countries. As shown in table 3, detection of only 13 unique infections and 35 'dual' HIV-1/HIV-2 infections (the majority of which are, in fact, believed to be unique HIV-1 infections) have been reported from just 3 countries (Brazil, USA, and Canada), figures dwarfed by almost 113 000 AIDS cases associated with HIV-1 reported from the Americas by June 1989 (WHO, 1989) and the estimated 1–1.5 million HIV-1 infections in the USA alone (CDC, 1989).

North America has acted as the focal point for the diffusion of HIV-1 within the Americas (Smallman-Raynor and Cliff, 1990a; 1990b). Diffusion corridors of HIV-2, shown in figure 10, stand in marked contrast. As with the spread of HIV-2 into Europe, there appear to be 2 principal poles: West and South Central Africa.

Within North America, an HIV-2 epidemic has yet to emerge. All 5 cases of unique HIV-2 infection reported from this part of the continent, 3 from Ontario, Canada (Neumann et al, 1988; 1989a; 1989b), 1 from

New Jersey, and 1 from New England, USA, (Ayanian et al, 1989; Weiss et al, 1988) have been West Africans.

The centrality of the Portuguese link in the global diffusion of HIV-2 recurs in South America. A clear picture of the HIV-2 epidemic in the former Portuguese colony of Brazil has yet to emerge. A total of 8 unique HIV-2 infections had been detailed, with a further 25 'dual' HIV-1/HIV-2 infections, by 30 July 1989 (table 3). Prevalence rates have been shown

Table 3. Number of HIV-2 and dual HIV-1/HIV-2 detections in the Americas.

Group	HIV-2	HIV-1/HIV-2
North America		
Canada[a]	3	0
USA[b]	2	10
South America		
Argentina[c]	0	0
Brazil[d]	8	25
Caribbean		
Guadeloupe[e]	0	0

[a] Neumann et al, 1988; 1989a; 1989b. [b] Ayanian et al, 1989; Weiss et al, 1988. [c] Bouzas et al, 1989. [d] Cortes et al, 1989a; 1989b; 1989c; 1989d; Santos-Ferreira et al, 1989; Sion et al, 1989; Veronesi et al, 1987. [e] Agius et al, 1989.

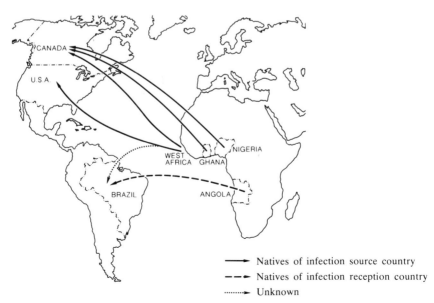

Figure 10. The diffusion of HIV-2 into the Americas. Sources: see table 3 and its footnotes.

to reach 4.1% among male transvestite prostitutes and 2% among female prostitutes (Santos-Ferreira et al, 1989), and reports of morbidity associated with HIV-2 have also been made in Rio de Janeiro (Sion et al, 1989). All detected infections have been in individuals of Brazilian origin and no direct African links are known. However, given the recently recognised extent of HIV-2 infection in Angola, a country historically linked to Brazil by Portugal, and the large numbers of Brazilians who have worked there, it is likely that this part of the African continent will eventually be shown to have acted as the diffusion pole for HIV-2 into the country (Cortes et al, 1989a).

7.2 HIV-2 in Asia
Few instances of serological analysis for the occurrence of HIV-2 infection in this continent have appeared to date, and the only evidence for infection with HIV-2 occurs in reports of 'dual' HIV-1/HIV-2 infection from southern India (Shanmugasundararaj et al, 1988). Whether these represent true dual infection is, however, doubtful. Nevertheless, it is possible that HIV-2 is spreading undetected on the continent. Neequaye et al (1986), for example, remark on the regularity of reports of Ghanaian prostitute contact with Koreans and Japanese in West Africa. Although limited work to date suggests no evidence of HIV-2 in Japan (Nakamura et al, 1987) further serological analysis is required in this part of the continent.

8 The global spread of HIV-2: a composite model
A time-dependent composite model of the global diffusion of HIV-2 based upon the foregoing reconstructions of spread is shown in figure 11. At time T_1, HIV-2 was restricted to a West African hearth, probably focused upon Guinea-Bissau (Clavel, 1987). The timing of the emergence of the virus is uncertain but could date back to the turn of the eighteenth century (Yokoyama et al, 1988) or before (Fukasawa et al, 1988).

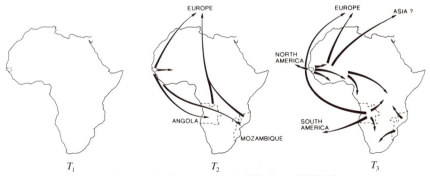

Figure 11. A composite model for the global diffusion of HIV-2.

At time T_2, HIV-2 began a restricted spread within West Africa as well as a movement to South Central Africa. The timing of this development is also uncertain, although reports have been made of HIV-2 in West African countries in the 1960s (Kawamura et al, 1989). Saimot et al (1987) and Botas et al (1989) record possible infections in Angola/ Mozambique in the late 1960s/early 1970s. At this time, HIV-2 also appears to have begun to diffuse into Portugal from both West and South Central Africa (for example, see Ancelle et al, 1987; Botas et al, 1989; Bryceson et al, 1988; Saimot et al, 1987).

At time T_3, in the 1980s, HIV-2 began to spread widely in West Africa, as well as disseminating into parts of Central and Southern Africa, Europe, the Americas, and possibly Asia from the principal West African diffusion pole and the subpole of Angola/Mozambique.

9 Conclusion

In this paper, we have attempted to outline the currently known geography of the AIDS virus, HIV-2, as presented in the medical literature. The picture is still highly fragmented; views concerning the virus are conflicting and figures relating to the occurrence of HIV-2 infection are dwarfed by the HIV-1 pandemic. However, it is already clear that the geographies of HIV-1 and HIV-2 are distinct: the major heartlands of the 2 viruses do not coincide and, consequently, the diffusion poles and corridors of spread of the 2 viruses differ.

A theme running through the international diffusion of HIV-2 is the Portuguese link. The early poles of infection [West Africa, Angola/ Mozambique (and Brazil?)], have been linked historically to Portugal and Portugal itself possesses the only developed HIV-2 epidemic in Europe.

These patterns suggest a number of research questions.

1 How may detailed analysis of the Portuguese link influence our understanding of the development of the global spread of HIV-1, given the uncertain evolutionary relationship between the 2 strains of HIV?

2 Now that distinct infection poles for HIV-2 are becoming established, how will its future international diffusion progress?

3 How will this diffusion differ from the patterns woven in the early stages of the HIV-1 pandemic?

4 Will the principal diffusion poles of HIV-2 shift with time so as to parallel those of HIV-1 as the virus establishes itself in the West?

5 How can the geographical variation in the spread of HIV-1 and HIV-2, coupled with the uncertain pathogenic potential and incubation period of the latter virus, be built into models to forecast the future spatial development of the global AIDS pandemic?

The global spread of HIV-1 and the associated AIDS pandemic caught the world by surprise. HIV-2, on the other hand, has a pandemic potential yet to be fully realised. HIV-2 is already in the early stages of developing subpoles of infection in Europe and Brazil that are creating a pattern of global diffusion for HIV-2 which is distinct from that for HIV-1, whose spread is dominated by the USA. This second AIDS virus offers a unqiue opportunity to observe, map, model, and forecast the development of an embryonic pandemic.

Acknowledgements. Dr F de la Cruz (Immunology Laboratory, Instituto Nacional de Saude, Maputo, Mozambique) provided information on the occurrence of HIV-2 infection in Southern and Central Africa, and Dr J Mann (World Health Organization Global Programme on AIDS, Geneva) supplied the WHO estimates of global AIDS cases to the end of 1988.

References
Abstracts of the V International Conference on AIDS are available from V International Conference on AIDS Secretariat, Kenness Canada Inc, 1010 Saint Catherine Street West, Suite 628, Montreal, Quebec H3B 1G7, Canada.

Agius G, Vaillant V, Dindinaud G, Bazillou M, Zagury J F, Castets M, 1989, "HTLV-I, HIV-1 and HIV-2 seroprevalences in Guadeloupe, French West Indies" *Proceedings* V International Conference on AIDS, Montreal, 4 – 9 June, abstract M.A.O.14

Ancelle R, Bletry O, Baglin A C, Brun-Vézinet F, Rey M A, Godeau P, 1987, "Long incubation period for HIV-2 infection" *Lancet* i 688 – 689

Andreasson P Å, Dias F, Teixeira Goudiaby J M, Nauclér A, Biberfield G, 1989, "HIV-2 infection in prenatal women in Guinea-Bissau" *Proceedings* V International Conference on AIDS, Montreal, 4 – 9 June, abstract M.G.P.16

Ayanian J, Maguire J, Kanki P, Marlink R, Mayer K, Essex M, 1989, "HIV-2 in New England" *Proceedings* V International Conference on AIDS, Montreal, 4 – 9 June, abstract M.B.P.200

Ayres L, Pista A, Benito-Garcia A, Furtado C, Avillez F, 1989, "Epidemiology of AIDS in Portugal" *Proceedings* V International Conference on AIDS, Montreal, 4 – 9 June, abstract M.A.P.82

Barré-Sinoussi F, Chermann J C, Rey F, Nugeyre M T, Chamaret S, Gruest J, Danguet C, Axler-Blin C, Vézinet-Brun F, Rouzioux C, Rozenbaum W, Montagnier L, 1983, "Isolation of a T-lymphotropic retrovirus from a patient at risk for acquired immune deficiency syndrome (AIDS)" *Science* **220** 868 – 871

Bayliss G J, Parry J V, Mortimer P P, 1988, "HIV-2 in Britain: no evidence, yet" *Lancet* **ii** 120

Berkley S, Okware S, Naamara W, 1989, "Surveillance for AIDS in Uganda" *AIDS* **3** 79 – 85

BHTD, 1986 – 87 *AIDS and Retroviruses Update* Bureau of Hygiene and Tropical Diseases, Keppel Street, London WC1E 7HT

BHTD, 1988, "Screening for HIV-2" *AIDS Newsletter* Bureau of Hygiene and Tropical Diseases, volume 3, number 833, page 3; available from BHTD, Keppel Street, London WC1E 7HT

Biesert L, Adamski M, Selb B, von Briesen H, Mix D A G, Roscher H E, Spiegelberg T, Valenteijn A, Schildwächter K, Sauer A, Doerr H W, Rübsamen-Waigmann H, 1988, "Origin and serological characteristics of HIV-2 cases diagnosed in West Germany" *AIDS-Forschung* **3** 329 – 332

Bigot A, Zohoun I, De Bruyere M, Latinne D, Burtonboy G, 1987, "Premiers cas de séropositivité anti-HIV-1 au Bénin" *La Presse Médicale* **16** 1102

Botas J, Tavores L, Carvalho C, Feliciano H, Antunes F, 1989, "HIV-2 infection. Some clinical and epidemiological aspects in Portugal" *Proceedings* V International Conference on AIDS, Montreal, 4 – 9 June, abstract M.A.P.77

Böttiger B, Palme I B, Da Costa J C, Dias L F, Biberfield G, 1988, "Prevalence of HIV-1 and HIV-2/HTLV-IV infections in Luanda and Cabinda, Angola" *Journal of Acquired Immune Deficiency Syndromes* **1** 8–12

Bouzas M B, Simon F, Muchinik G, Picchio G, Brun-Vézinet F, Mathov I, 1989, "Absence of HIV-2-infection in haemophilia in Buenos Aires" *Proceedings* V International Conference on AIDS, Montreal, 4–9 June, abstract Th.B.P.3

Brücker G, Brun-Vézinet F, Rosenheim M, Rey M A, Katlama C, Gentilini M, 1987, "HIV-2 infection in 2 homosexual men in France" *Lancet* **i** 223

Brun-Vézinet F, Katlama C, Roulot D, Lenoble L, Alizon M, Madjar J J, Rey M A, Griard P M, Yeni P, Clavel F, Gadelle S, Harzic M, 1987, "Lymphadenopathy-associated virus type 2 in AIDS and AIDS-related complex. Clinical and virological features in 4 patients" *Lancet* **i** 128–132

Bryceson A, Tomkins A, Ridley D, Warhurst D, Goldstone A, Bayliss G, Toswill J, Parry J, 1988, "HIV-2-associated AIDS in the 1970s" *Lancet* **ii** 221

Buttò S, Verani P, Titti F, Rezza G, Sernicola L, Rossi G B, 1988, "Simultaneous seropositivity to HIV-1 and HIV-2 in Italian drug abusers" *AIDS* **2** 139–140

Cadeo G P, Corda L, Pizzocolo G, Albertini A, Carosi G, 1989, "HIV-2 in Italy: no evidence, yet" *Proceedings* V International Conference on AIDS, Montreal, 4–9 June, abstract M.A.P.78

Cardoso J, Avillez F, Santos I, Pista A, Ayres L, 1989, "Prevalence of HIV-1 and HIV-2 antibodies in individuals attending a clinic for STD. A two year follow-up" *Proceedings* V International Conference on AIDS, Montreal, 4–9 June, abstract M.A.P.86

CDC, 1989, "AIDS and human immunodeficiency virus infection in the United States: 1988 update", Centers for Disease Control *Morbidity and Mortality Weekly Report* **38** (supplement 4) 1–38

Chakrabarti L, Guyader M, Alizon M, Daniel M D, Desrosiers R C, Tiollais P, Sonigo P, 1987, "Sequence of simian immunodeficiency virus from macaques and its relationship to other human and simian retroviruses" *Nature* **328** 543–547

Chevallier P, Ritter J, Andriamampithantona E, Sepetjan M, 1989, "Prevalence des infections par le virus HIV1, HIV2 et HTLV1 dans la region de Tananarive, Madagascar" *Proceedings* V International Conference on AIDS, Montreal, 4–9 June, abstract M.G.P.7

Chin J, Mann J, 1989, "Global surveillance and forecasting of AIDS" *Bulletin of the World Health Organization* **67** 1–7

Clavel F, 1987, "HIV-2: the West African AIDS virus" *AIDS* **1** 135–140

Clavel F, Guétard D, Brun-Vézinet F, Chamaret S, Rey M A, Santos-Ferreira M O, Laurent A G, Dauguet C, Katlama C, Rouzioux C, Klatzmann D, Champalimaud J L, Montagnier L, 1986, "Isolation of a new human retrovirus from West African patients with AIDS" *Science* **233** 343–346

Clavel F, Mansinho K, Chamaret S, Guétard D, Favier V, Nina J, Santos-Ferreira M O, Champalimaud J L, Montagnier L, 1987, "Human immundeficiency virus Type 2 infection associated with AIDS in West Africa" *New England Journal of Medicine* **316** 1180–1185

Coffin J, Haase A, Levy J A, Montagnier L, Oroszlan S, Teich N, Temin H, Toyoshima K, Varmus H, Vogt P, Weiss R, 1986, "What to call the AIDS virus" *Nature* **321** 10

Constantine D, Fox E, Rodier G, Abbatte E, 1989, "Monitoring for HIV-1, HIV-2, HTLV-1 sero-progression and sero-conversion" *Proceedings* V International Conference on AIDS, Montreal, 4–9 June, abstract B.538

Contreras G, Garcia A, Vallhonrat E, Varela J M, Peres Alvarez L, Najera R, 1989, "Prevalence of different retroviruses in Spanish intravenous drug users during 1.987 – 1.988. Clinical findings of seropositives" *Proceedings* V International Conference on AIDS, Montreal, 4 – 9 June, abstract A.576

Cortes E, Detels R, Aboulafia D, Li X L, Moudgil T, Alam M, Bonecker C, Gonzaga A, Oyafuso L, Tondo M, Boite C, Hammershlak N, Capitani C, Slamon D J, Ho D D, 1989a, "HIV-1, HIV-2 and HTLV-1 infection in high risk groups in Brazil" *New England Journal of Medicine* **320** 953 – 958

Cortes E, Detels R, Slamon D, Aboulafia D, Li X L, Ho D D, 1989b, "Study of HIV-1, HIV-2, and HTLV-1 in homosexuals in Brazil" *Proceedings* V International Conference on AIDS, Montreal, 4 – 9 June, abstract M.G.P.12

Cortes E, Detels R, Slamon D, Aboulafia D, Li X L, Ho D D, 1989c, "Study of HIV-1, HIV-2 and HTLV-1 in female prostitutes in Brazil" *Proceedings* V International Conference on AIDS, Montreal, 4 – 9 June, abstract M.G.P.13

Cortes E, Detels R, Slamon D, Aboulafia D, Li X L, Ho D D, 1989d, "Seroprevalence of HIV-1, HIV-2 and HTLV-1 in Brazilian bisexual males" *Proceedings* V International Conference on AIDS, Montreal, 4 – 9 June, abstract M.G.P.14

Cour M I, Palau L, Fernández Contreras E, Perezagua C, Ladrón de Guevara J, 1989, "HIV-1, HIV-2 and HTLV-1 in Spanish inmates" *AIDS* **3** 320 – 321

Couroucé A M, 1987, "HIV-2 in blood donors and in different groups in France" *Lancet* **i** 1151

Couroucé A M, and The "Retrovirus" Study Group of the French Society of Blood Transfusion, 1988, "A prospective study of HIV-2 prevalence in France" *AIDS* **2** 261 – 265

CS/BHTD, 1988 – 89 *Current AIDS Literature* prepared by Current Science in association with Bureau of Hygiene and Tropical Diseases; available from Current Science, 34 – 42 Cleveland Street, London W1P 5FB

DeCock K M, Porter A, Moreau J, Diaby L, Odehouri K, Heyward W, 1989, "Sentinel site surveillance for AIDS in Abidjan, Côte D'Ivoire" *Proceedings* V International Conference on AIDS, Montreal, 4 – 9 June, abstract M.G.O.27

de la Cruz F, Barreto J, Palha de Sousa C, Barquet L, 1989, "HIV in Mozambique. A general overview" *Proceedings* V International Conference on AIDS, Montreal, 4 – 9 June, abstract Th.G.P.22

Denis F, Barin F, Gershy-Damet G, Rey J L, Lhuillier M, Mounier M, Leonard G, Sangaré A, Goudeau A, M'Boup S, Essex M, Kanki P, 1987, "Prevalence of human T-lymphotropic retroviruses Type III (HIV) and Type IV in Ivory Coast" *Lancet* **i** 408 – 411

Dufoort G, Couroucé A M, Ancelle-Park R, Bletry O, 1988, "No clinical signs 14 years after HIV-2 transmission via blood transfusion" *Lancet* **ii** 510

Essex M, 1989, "The origins of human retroviruses" *Proceedings* V International Conference on AIDS, Montreal, 4 – 9 June, abstract T.C.O.23

Essex M, Kanki P J, 1988, "The origins of the AIDS virus" *Scientific American* **259** 44 – 51

Essien E, Saliu I, 1989, "HIV-2 seroprevalence in different groups tested in University College Hospital, Ibadan, Nigeria" *Proceedings* V International Conference on AIDS, Montreal, 4 – 9 June, abstract M.B.P.158

Evans L A, Moreau J, Odehouri K, Legg H, Barboza A, Cheng-Mayer C, Ley J A, 1988a, "Characterization of a noncytopathic HIV-2 strain with unusual effects on CD4 expression" *Science* **240** 1522 – 1525

Evans L A, Moreau J, Odehouri K, Seto D, Thomson-Honnebier G, Legg H, Barboza A, Cheng-Meyer C, Levy J A, 1988b, "Simultaneous isolation of HIV-1 and HIV-2 from an AIDS patient" *Lancet* **ii** 1389 – 1391

Ferroni P, Tagger A, Lazzarin A, Moroni M, 1987, "HIV-1 and HIV-2 infections
    in Italian AIDS/ARC patients" *Lancet* **i** 869–870
Fleming A F, 1988, "AIDS in Africa: an update" *AIDS-Forschung* **3** 116–134
Foucault-Fretz C, Gluckman J C, Foumel J J, Kourouma K, Diallo P, Diallo K,
    1989, "Double HIV1 and HIV2 seropositivity in Guinea" *Proceedings* V
    International Conference on AIDS, Montreal, 4–9 June, abstract T.G.P.28
Fountouli P, Karnela A, Bertoli A M, Ammar A, Malliaraki-Pinetidou E, Jasmin C,
    Georgoulias V, 1989, "Detection of antibodies against HIV-2 proteins in HIV-1
    seropositive subjects from France and Greece" *Proceedings* V International
    Conference on AIDS, Montreal, 4–9 June, abstract M.A.P.80
Fukasawa M, Miura T, Hasegawa S, Tsujimoto H, Miki K, Kitamura T, Hayami M,
    1988, "Sequence of simian immunodeficiency virus from African green
    monkey, a new member of the HIV/SIV group" *Nature* **333** 457–461
Fultz P N, McClure H M, Anderson D C, Swenson R B, Anand R, Srinivasan A,
    1986, "Isolation of a T-lymphotropic retrovirus from naturally infected sooty
    mangabey monkeys (*Cercocebus atys*)" *Proceedings of the National Academy of
    Sciences USA* **83** 5286–5290
Fultz P N, Switzer W M, Schable C A, Desrosiers R C, Silva D P, McCormick J B,
    1988, "Seroprevalence of HIV-1 and HIV-2 in Guinea-Bissau in 1980" *AIDS*
    2 129–132
Gallo R C, Salahuddin S Z, Popvic M, Shearer G M, Kaplan M, Haynes B F,
    Palker T J, Redfield R, Oleske J, Safai B, White G, Foster P, Markham P D,
    1984, "Frequent detection and isolation of cytopathic retroviruses (HTLV-III)
    from patients with AIDS and at risk of AIDS" *Science* **224** 500–503
Georges A J, Georges-Courbet M C, Slaun D, Martin P M V, Barré-Sinoussi F,
    Coulaud X, Chouaid E, 1988, "Isolation of HIV-2 in Central Africa from
    AIDS patient and her symptom-free partner" *Lancet* **i** 188–189
Georgoulias V, Fountouli D, Karvela-Agelakis A, Komis G, Malliaraki-
    Pinetidou E, Antoniadis G, Samakidis K, Kondakis X, Papapertropoulou M,
    Zoumbos N, Axenidou O, Makris K, Sonidis G, 1988, "HIV-1 and HIV-2
    double infection in Greece" *Annals of Internal Medicine* **108** 155
Gody M, Ouattara S A, de-Thé G, 1988, "Clinical experience of AIDS in relation
    to HIV-1 and HIV-2 infection in a rural hospital in Ivory Coast, West Africa"
    AIDS **2** 433–436
Gonda M A, Brau M J, Clements J E, Pyper J M, Wong-Staal F, Gallo R C,
    Gilden R V, 1986, "Human T-cell lymphotropic virus type III shares sequence
    homology with a family of pathogenic Lentiviruses" *Proceedings of the National
    Academy of Sciences USA* **83** 4007–4011
Gottlieb M S, Schroff R, Schanker H M, Weisman J D, Fan P T, Wolf R A,
    Saxon A S, 1981 *Pneumocystis carinii* pneumonia and mucosal candidiasis in
    previously healthy homosexual men: evidence of a new acquired cellular
    immunodeficiency" *New England Journal of Medicine* **305** 1425–1431
Gresenguet G, Belec L, Gonzales J P, Georges A J, 1988, "Sero-surveillance de
    l'infection HIV en zones rurales de Republique Centrafricaine: bilan 1985–87"
    Médecine d'Afrique Noire **35** 243–246
Grote J, 1988, "Bovine visna virus and the origin of HIV" *Journal of the Royal
    Society of Medicine* **81** 620
Heath R B, Grint P C A, Hardiman A E, 1988, "Anonymous testing of women
    attending antenatal clinics for evidence of infection with HIV" *Lancet* **i** 1394
Hirsch V M, Murphey-Corb M, Johnson P R, 1989, "SIV from sooty mangabey
    monkeys: an African primate Lentivirus closely related to HIV-2" *Proceedings*
    V International Conference on AIDS, Montreal, 4–9 June, abstract T.C.O.43

Horsburgh C R Jr, Holmberg S D, 1988, "The global distribution of human immunodeficiency virus type 2 (HIV-2) infection" *Transfusion* **28** 192–195

Hrdy D B, 1987, "Cultural practices contributing to the transmission of human immunodeficiency virus in Africa" *Reviews of Infectious Diseases* **9** 1109–1119

Hymes K B, Cheung T, Greene J B, Prose N S, Marcus A, Ballard H, William D C, Laubenstein L J, 1981, "Kaposi's sarcoma in homosexual men—a report of eight cases" *Lancet* **ii** 598–600

Ishikawa K, Tsujimoto H, Nakai M, Mingle J A A, Osei-Kwasi M, Aggrey S E, Nettey V B A, Afoakwa S N, Fukasawa M, Kodama T, Kawamura M, Hayami M, 1988, "Isolation and characterization of HIV-2 from an AIDS patient in Ghana" *AIDS* **2** 383–388

Kanki P J, 1987, "West African human retroviruses related to STLV-III" *AIDS* **1** 141–145

Kanki P J, Allan J, Barin F, Redfiled R, Clumeck N, Quinn T, Mowovondi F, Thiry L, Burny A, Zagury D, Petat E, Kocheleff P, Pascal K, Lausen I, Fredericksen B, Craighead J, M'Boup S, Denis F, Curran J W, Mann J, Francis H, Albaum M, Travers K, McLane M F, Lee T H, Essex M, 1987, "Absence of antibodies to HIV-2/HTLV-4 in six Central African nations" *AIDS Research and Human Retroviruses* **3** 317–322

Kanki P J, Barin F, M'Boup S, Allan J S, Romet-Lemonne J L, Marlink R, McLane M F, Lee T H, Arbeille B, Denis F, Essex M, 1986, "New human T-lymphotropic retrovirus related to simian T-lymphotropic virus type III (STLV IIIagm)" *Science* **232** 238–243

Kanki P, M'Boup S, Romieu I, Marlink R, Siby T, Essex M, 1989, "Epidemiology of HIV-2 in female prostitutes in Senegal" *Proceedings* V International Conference on AIDS, Montreal, 4–9 June, abstract M.A.O.15

Kaptue L, Zekeng L, Ngu K, Ouattara A, Monny-Lobe M, Salla R, 1989, "First case of HIV1/HIV2 infection in Cameroon" *Proceedings* V International Conference on AIDS, Montreal, 4–9 June, abstract A.573

Kawamura M, Yamazakai S, Ishikawa K, Kwofie T B, Tsujimoto H, Hayami M, 1989, "HIV2 in West Africa in 1966" *Lancet* **i** 385

Kestler H W III, Li Y, Waidu Y M, Bulter C V, Ochs M F, Jaenel G, King N W, Daniel M D, Desrosiers R C, 1988, "Comparison of simian immunodeficiency isolates" *Nature* **331** 619–621

Kingman S, 1987, "Equal spread in Norway" *New Scientist* **1570** 23

Kong L I, Lee S W, Kappes J C, Parkin J S, Decker D, Hoxie J A, Hahn B H, Shaw G M, 1988, "West African HIV-2 related human retrovirus with attenuated cytopathicity" *Science* **240** 1525–1529

Konotey-Ahulu F I D, 1989, "HIV-2 in West Africa" *Lancet* **i** 553

Kosia A, Kargbo T, Thorlie I, Monsaray N, Makiu E, Kanu J, 1989, "Prevalence of HIV seropositivity among STD patients in Freetown—Sierra Leone" *Proceedings* V International Conference on AIDS, Montreal, 4–9 June, abstract W.G.P.16

Kroegel C, Hess zum Büschenfelde G, Meyer K H, 1987, "Routes of HIV-2 transmission in Western Europe" *Lancet* **i** 1150

Kvinesdal B B, Hojiyng N, Molbak K, Aaby P, 1989, "Vertical transmission of HIV-2; lack of evidence" *Proceedings* V International Conference on AIDS, Montreal, 4–9 June, abstract G.517

Lancet, 1988, "HIV-2 in perspective" *Lancet* **i** 1027–1028

Lecatsas G, Joubert J J, Schutte C H J, Taylor M B, Swanevelder C, 1989, "Peak prevalence of HIV in Namibian teenagers" *Proceedings* V International Conference on AIDS, Montreal, 4–9 June, abstract Th.H.P.19

Le Guenno B, Sarthou J L, 1989, "Immunological parameters of HIV-1 and HIV-2 seropositives" *Proceedings* V International Conference on AIDS, Montreal, 4 – 9 June, abstract Th.B.P.151

Le Guenno B, Jean P, Pegbhini M, Griffet P, Seignot P, Barabe P, Ball M D, Montalegre A, N'Diaye B, Guirard M, Arborio M, Jouan A, Sarthou J L, 1987a, "Increasing HIV-2-associated AIDS in Senegal" *Lancet* ii 972 – 973

Le Guenno B, Jouan A, Arborio M, 1987b, "HIV-2 responsible for AIDS cases in Senegal" *Annales de l'Institute Pasteur: Virologie* 138E 397 – 399

Leinikki P, Hakulinen J, Kantanen M L, Brummer-Korvenkontio H, 1989, "Surveillance of HIV-2 infections by ELISA using HIV-1 and HIV-2 specific synthetic peptides" *Proceedings* V International Conference on AIDS, Montreal, 4 – 9 June, abstract A.509

Levy J A, Mitra G, Mozen M M, 1984, "Recovery and inactivation of infectious retrovirus added to factor VIII concentrates" *Lancet* ii 722 – 723

Li Y, Naidu Y M, Kestler H W, Fultz P, Daniel M D, Desrosier R C, 1989, "SIVsmm, a possible progenitor of HIV-2 and SIVmac" *Proceedings* V International Conference on AIDS, Montreal, 4 – 9 June, abstract Th.C.P.58

Lisse I, Poulsen A G, Aaby P, Kvinesdal B B, Molbak K, Dias F, Lauritzen E, 1989, "HIV-2 infection and immunodeficiency" *Proceedings* V International Conference on AIDS, Montreal, 4 – 9 June, abstract Th.B.P.156

Lourenço M H, Chen T, Octávio F, Santos-Ferreira M O, Matos-Almeida M J, Azevedo Pereira J M, 1989, "Incidence of HBV markers and HIV antibodies in blood donors in Luanda and Dundo, People's Republic of Angola" *Proceedings* V International Conference on AIDS, Montreal, 4 – 9 June, abstract A.511

Loveday C, Pomeroy L, Weller I V D, Quirk J, Hawkins A, Williams H, Smith A, Williams P, Tedder R S, Adler M W, 1989, "Human immunodeficiency viruses in patients attending a sexually transmitted disease clinic in London 1982 – 7" *British Medical Journal* 298 419 – 422

Lowenstine L J, Pederson N C, Higgins J, Pallis K C, Uydea A, Preston M, Lerche N W, Munn R J, Gardner M B, 1986, "Seroepidemiologic survey of cpative Old-World primates for antibodies to human and simian retroviruses, and isolation of a Lentivirus from sooty mangabeys (*Cercocebus atys*)" *International Journal of Cancer* 38 563 – 574

Lui K J, Darrow D, Rutherford G W III, 1988, "A model-based estimate for the mean incubation period for AIDS in homosexual men" *Science* 240 1333 – 1335

Lui K J, Lawrence D N, Morgan W M, 1986, "A model-based approach for estimating the mean incubation period of transfusion-associated acquired immunodeficiency syndrome" *Proceedings of the National Academy of Sciences USA* 83 3051 – 3055

Lyons S F, Clausen L, Schoub B D, 1988a, "HIV-2-induced AIDS in southern Africa" *AIDS* 2 406 – 407

Lyons S F, Smith A N, McGillivray G M, Schoub B D, 1988b, "HIV-2 infection in South Africa" *Transactions of the Society of Tropical Medicine and Hygiene* 12 757

Lyons S F, McGillivray G, Schoub B D, Smith A N, Chausen L, 1989, "AIDS caused by HIV-2 in southern Africa" *Proceedings* V International Conference on AIDS, Montreal, 4 – 9 June, abstract M.A.P.83

Mabey D C W, Tedder R S, Hughes A S B, Corrah P T, Goodison S J F, O'Connor T, Shenton F C, Lucas S B, Whittle H C, Greenwood B M, 1988, "Human retroviral infections in the Gambia: prevalence and clinical features" *British Medical Journal* 296 83 – 86

McClure M, Schulz T F, 1989, "Origin of HIV" *British Medical Journal* **298** 1267-1268

Malkin J E, Prazuck T H, Simonnet F, Traore E, Tiendrebeogo H, Dublanchet A, Deborne B, Vincent-Ballereua F, Lafaix C H, 1989, "Tuberculose et infection a VIH a Bobo-Dioulasso (Burkina Faso)" *Proceedings* V International Conference on AIDS, Montreal, 4-9 June, abstract M.G.P.26

Mann J M, Chin J, Piot P, Quinn T, 1988, "The international epidemiology of AIDS" *Scientific American* **259** 60-69

Mannuci P M, Gringeri A, Bianchi A, 1989, "Different epidemiology of HIV infection in haemophiliacs (H) from three European countries" *Proceedings* V International Conference on AIDS, Montreal, 4-9 June, abstract M.A.P.44

Marlink R, Thior I, Siby T, N'Doye L, Kanki P, Romieu I, 1989, "Observations on the natural history of HIV-2" *Proceedings* V International Conference on AIDS, Montreal, 4-9 June, abstract M.A.O.13

Martegani R, Magni E, Incarbone C, Parini A, Fiori G P, Montanari M, Sampietro C, Torre D, Dietz A, 1988, "Sieroepidemiologia di HIV-1 e HIV-2 in tossicodipendenti" *Giornale di Malattie Infettive e Parassitarie* **40** 685-687

Masur H, Michelis M A, Greene J B, Onorato I, Vande Stouwe R A, Holzman R S, Mormser G, Brettman L, Lange M, Murray H W, Cunningham-Rundles S, 1981, "An outbreak of community-acquired *Pneumocystis carinii* pneumonia: initial manifestation of cellular immune dysfunction" *New England Journal of Medicine* **305** 1431-1438

Matos-Almeida M J M, Santos-Ferreira M O, Lourenço M H, Chen T, Azevedo Pereira J M, 1989, "HIV-1 and HIV-2 serological survey in Luanda Norte, Northeastern province of Republica Popular de Angola" *Proceedings* V International Conference on AIDS, Montreal, 4-9 June, abstract M.G.P.2

M'Boup S, N'Doye I, Samb A, Siby T, Boye C B, Sangaré L, 1989, "Problematique de l'infection HIV-2: exemple du Senegal" *Proceedings* V International Conference on AIDS, Montreal, 4-9 June, abstract T.G.P.26

Medley G F, Anderson R M, Cox D R, Billard L, 1987, "Incubation period of AIDS in patients infected by blood transfusion" *Nature* **328** 719-721

Mertens T H, Tondorf G, Siebolds M, Kruppenbacher J P, Shretha S M, Mauff G, Gürtler L, Eggers H J, 1989, "Epidemiology of HIV and hepatitis B virus (HBV) in selected African and Asian populations" *Infection* **17** 4-7

Mintz E, Peale R, Mathur S K, Prince A, Brotman B, 1988, "A serologic study of HIV infection in Liberia" *Journal of Acquired Immune Deficiency Syndromes* **1** 67-68

Modrow S, Wolf H, Löwer J, Kurth R, 1987, "Verwandtschaftliche Beziehung von HIV-isolaten zu anderen vertretern der Lentivirusgruppe" *AIDS-Forschung* **2** 679-688

Mohammed I, Harry T O, Nasidi A, 1989, "HIV-2 in West Africa in 1966" *Lancet* **1** 1137

Montagnier L, 1988, "Origin and evolution of HIVs and their role in AIDS pathogenesis" *Journal of Acquired Immune Deficiency Syndromes* **1** 517-520

Moore A, Le Baron R D, 1986, "The case for a Haitian origin of the AIDS epidemic", in *The Social Dimensions of AIDS: Method and Theory* Eds D A Feldman, T M Johnson (Praeger, New York) pp 77-93

Mulder C, 1988, "A case of mistaken non-identity" *Nature* **331** 562-563

Murphey-Corb M, Martin L N, Rangan S R S, Baskin G B, Gormus B J, Wolf R H, Andes W A, West M, Montelaro R C, 1986, "Isolation of an HTLV-III-related retrovirus from macaques with simian AIDS and its possible origin in asymptomatic mangabeys" *Nature* **321** 435-437

Nakamura K, Yoshida Y, Ando T, Yamazaki K, Ohnuki N, Ito T, Yano K, Sekine S, Hayashi Y, Sinkai T, Hori M, Teragama T, Yabuuchi K, Miki T, Ishkawa K, Hayami M, Ohashi M, 1987, "A serological survey for human immunodeficiency virus types 1 and 2 of individuals who visited health centres in Tokyo" *Japanese Journal of Medical Science and Biology* **40** 159-164

Nauclér A, Andreasson P Å, Mendes C, Thorstensson R, Biberfield G, 1989, "HIV-2-associated AIDS and HIV-2 seroprevalence in Bissau, Guinea-Bissau" *Journal of Acquired Immune Deficiency Syndromes* **2** 88-93

Neequaye A R, Neequaye J, Mingle J A, Ofori Adjei D, 1986, "Preponderance of females with AIDS in Ghana" *Lancet* **ii** 978

Neequaye A R, Osei L, Mingle J A A, Ankra-Badu G, Bentsi C, Asamoah-Adu A, Neequaye J E, 1988, "Dynamics of human immune deficiency virus (HIV) cpidemic—the Ghanaian experience", in *The Global Impact of AIDS* Eds A F Fleming, M Carballo, D W FitzSimons, M R Bailey, J M Mann (Alan R Liss, New York) pp 9-15

Neumann P W, Lepine D, Woodside M, Levesque J, Frenette S, O'Shaughnessy M V, D'Souza I, Major C, Gregory B, Bond V, Strune G, McLaughlin B, 1988, "HIV-2 infection detected in Canada" *Canada Diseases Weekly Report* **14** 125-126

Neumann P W, O'Shaughnessy M V, Lepine D, D'Souza I, Major C, McLaughlin B, 1989a, "Laboratory diagnosis of the first cases of HIV-2 infection in Canada" *Canadian Medical Association Journal* **140** 125-128

Neumann P W, O'Shaughnessy M V, Lepine D, D'Souza I, Major C, McLaughlin B, 1989b, "HIV infection in Canada" *Proceedings* V International Conference on AIDS, Montreal, 4-9 June, abstract T.B.P.106

Odehouri K, De Cock K, Colebunders R, Porter A, Adjorlolo G, Heyward W, 1989, "Clinical manifestations of HIV-1 and HIV-2 infections in Abidjan, Cote D'Ivoire" *Proceedings* V International Conference on AIDS, Montreal, 4-9 June, abstract T.B.O.10

Oelman B, Wilkins H A, Hughes A, Whittle H, Jaiteh K O, Cham M K, 1989, "The epidemiology of HIV-1 and HIV-2 in the Gambia, West Africa" *Proceedings* V International Conference on AIDS, Montreal, 4-9 June, abstract T.G.P.30

Ouattara S A, Chotard J, Meite M, Selly-Essis A M, de-Thé G, 1986, "Retrovirus infections (LAV/HTLV-III) and HTLV-I in Ivory Coast, West Africa" *Annales de l'Institute Pasteur: Virologie* **137E** 303-310

Ouattara S A, Gody M, Rioche M, Sangaré A, Meité M, Akran Y, Aron Y, Sanogo I, Ouattara D, Saraka K, Sombo M, Cabennes R, de-Thé G, 1988, "Blood transfusions and HIV infections (HIV1, HIV2/LAV2) in Ivory Coast" *Journal of Tropical Medicine and Hygiene* **91** 212-215

Ouattara S A, Meité M, Cot M C, de-Thé G, 1989, "Compared prevalence of infections by HIV-1 and HIV-2 during a 2-year period in suburban and rural areas of Ivory Coast" *Journal of Acquired Immune Deficiency Syndromes* **2** 94-99

Ousséini H, Pécarrère J, Madras R, Cénac A, Seyni M, Delevoux M, 1989, "Le SIDA en républic du Niger" *La Presse Médicale* **18** 1298

Palha de Sousa C, Barreto J, de la Cruz J, Barquet L, Bomba A, Chamera L, Costa E, Faustino H, Mondlane C, 1989, "The influence of war on HIV epidemic in Mozambique" *Proceedings* V International Conference on AIDS, Montreal, 4-9 June, unlisted poster presentation; paper available from C Palha de Sousa, Immunology Laboratory, Instituto Nacional de Saude, Maputo, Mozambique

Pepin J, Egboga A, Alonso P, Gaye I, Whittle H, Wilkins A, 1989, "Prevalence
    and correlates of retroviral infections among prostitutes working in Gambia"
    Proceedings V International Conference on AIDS, Montreal, 4-9 June,
    abstract T.G.P.32
Peterlin B M, Luciw P A, 1988, "Molecular biology of HIV" *AIDS* 2 (supplement 1)
    S29-S40
Pintus A, Piras S, Contu L, Pitzus F, 1989, "HIV-2 infection in Sardinia"
    Proceedings V International Conference on AIDS, Montreal, 4-9 June,
    abstract A.634
Piot P, Plummer F A, Mhalu F S, Lamboray J L, Chin J, Mann J M, 1988,
    "AIDS: an international perspective" *Science* 239 573-579
Piot P, Taelman H, Minlangu K B, Mbendi N, Ndangi K, Kalambayi K, Bridts C,
    Quinn T C, Feinsod F M, Wobin O, Mazrbo P, Stevens W, Mitchell S,
    McCormick J B, 1984, "Acquired immunodeficiency syndrome in a
    heterosexual population in Zaire" *Lancet* ii 65-69
Pokrovskii V V, Suvorova Z K, Mangushev T N, 1988, "Type 2 human
    immunodeficiency virus (HIV-2) infection in the USSR" *Zhurnal Mikrobiologii
    Epidemiologii i Immunobiologii* 10 18-20
Poulsen A G, Kvinesdal B B, Aaby P, Frederiksen K, Molbak K, Dias F, 1989a,
    "No evidence of vertical transmission of HIV-2 in Bissau" *Proceedings* V
    International Conference on AIDS, Montreal, 4-9 June, abstract T.G.P.31
Poulsen A G, Kvinesdal B, Aaby P, Molbak K, Frederiksen K, Dias F, Lauritzen E,
    1989b, "Prevalence of and mortality from human immunodeficiency virus
    type 2 in Bissau, West Africa" *Lancet* i 827-831
Rees M, 1987, "The sombre view of AIDS" *Nature* 362 343-345
Rey M A, Girard P M, Harzic M, Madjar J J, Brun-Vézinet F, Saimot A G,
    1987, "HIV-1 and HIV-2 double infection in French homosexual male with
    AIDS-related complex (Paris, 1985)" *Lancet* i 388-389
Rey F, Salaun D, Lesbordes J L, Gadelle S, Ollivier-Henry F, Barré-Sinoussi F,
    Chermann J C, Georges A J, 1986, "HIV-1 and HIV-II double infection in
    Central African Republic" *Lancet* ii 1391-1392
Ricard D, M'Boup S, Denis F, Essex M, 1989, "Coinfections HIV-2/HTLV-1
    dans un groupe de sujects a risque au Senegal" *Proceedings* V International
    Conference on AIDS, Montreal, 4-9 June, abstract T.G.P.29
Romieu I, Marlink R, M'Boup S, Kanki P J, Hernandez M, Essex M, 1989,
    "HIV-2 link to AIDS" *Proceedings* V International Conference on AIDS,
    Montreal, 4-9 June, abstract T.G.P.27
Rouzioux C, Burgard M, Courgnaud V, Bréchot C, Gazengel C, Berche P, 1989,
    "Isolation of HIV in a HIV-1-HIV-2 dual seroconverted child infected by
    blood transfusion in 1984 in France: characterization with PCR" *Proceedings* V
    International Conference on AIDS, Montreal, 4-9 June, abstract Th.C.P.21
Rübsamen-Waigmann H, Adamski M, Esser R, Heichsner C, Kühnel H,
    von Briesen H, Dietrich U, 1989, "Two West African isolates of HIV-2 with
    marked tropism for macrophages, one of which is highly divergent and genetically
    equidistant between HIV-2rod and SIVmac" *Proceedings* V International
    Conference on AIDS, Montreal, 4-9 June, abstract Th.C.O.4
Rwandan HIVSG, 1989, "Nationwide community-based serological survey of
    HIV-1 and other human retrovirus infections in a Central African country",
    Rwandan HIV Seroprevalence Group *Lancet* i 941-943
Saal F, Sidibe S, Alves-Cardoso E, Terrinha A, Gessain A, Poiot Y, Montagnier L,
    Peries J, 1987, "Anti-HIV-2 serological screening in Portuguese populations
    native from or having had close contact with Africa" *AIDS Research and
    Human Retroviruses* 3 341-342

Sabatier R, 1988 *Blaming Others: Prejudice, Race and Worldwide AIDS* (PANOS Institute, London)

Saimot A G, Couland J P, Mechati D, Matherson S, Dazza M C, Rey M A, Brun-Vézinet F, Leibowitch J, 1987, "HIV-2/LAV-2 in Portuguese man with AIDS (Paris, 1978) who had served in Angola 1968-74" *Lancet* **i** 688

Sangaré L, Kanki P, Soudré R, Tiendrebéogo H, M'Boup S, Essex M, 1989, "Statut serologique d'une population de prostituees doublement aux HIV-1 et HIV-2 au Burkina Faso" *Proceedings* V International Conference on AIDS, Montreal, 4-9 June, abstract Th.G.O.26

Santos-Ferreira M O, Mazza C, Lourenço M H, Focaccia R, Veronesi R, 1989, "HIV-2 infection in female and male Brazilian prostitute groups" *Proceedings* V International Conference on AIDS, Montreal, 4-9 June, abstract M.A.P.84

Scasso A, Moretti A, Greco F, Gambardella L, 1988, "L'infezione da HIV-2 in Toscuna: risultati preliminari di una indagine epidemiologica" *Giornale di Malattie Infettive e Parassitarie* **40** 526-529

Schmidt B L, Gschnalt F, Mayer F, Hutterer J, Bonekowich F, Schulz T F, Dierich M, 1989, "Cross reaction between HIV-1 and HIV-2 or double infection" *Proceedings* V International Conference on AIDS, Montreal, 4-9 June, abstract W.B.P.98

Schoub B D, Smith A N, Lyons S F, Johnson S, Martin D J, McGillivray G, Padayachee G N, Naidoo S, Fischer E L, Hurwitz H S, 1988, "Epidemiological considerations of the present status and future growth of the acquired immunodeficiency syndrome epidemic in South Africa" *South African Medical Journal* **74** 153-157

Shanmugasundararaj A, Williams J, Veluchamy V, Pothiraju Y, Chitra A, 1988, "Seropositivity for HIV-2 in Maduri, Tamil Nadu, India" *Virus Information Exchange Newsletter* **5** 132

Siegal F P, Lopez C, Hammer G S, Brown A E, Kornfield S J, Gold J, Hassett J, Hirschmann Z, Cunningham-Rundles C, Adelsberg B R, Parham D M, Siegal M, Cunningham-Rundles S, Armstrong D, 1981, "Severe acquired immunodeficiency in male homosexuals, manifested by chronic perianal ulcerative herpes simplex lesions" *New England Journal of Medicine* **305** 1439-1444

Simon F, Peeters M, Andrade D, Theobald S, Maiga Y, Cot M C, Brun-Vézinet F, 1989a, "Geographical variation in cross-reactivity of HIV-2 sera on HIV-1 assay" *Proceedings* V International Conference on AIDS, Montreal, 4-9 June, abstract C.745

Simon F, Puel J, Hammer R, Courgnaud V, Kirpach P, Brun-Vézinet F, 1989b, "HIV-2 infection in 2 European haemophiliac patients" *Proceedings* V International Conference on AIDS, Montreal, 4-9 June, abstract T.B.P.109

Sion F S, Sereno A B, Krebs J W, Gonçalves R S, Quinhoes E P, Weniger B G, Perez M A, Santos E A, Ramos Filho C F, Valiante P M, Ismael C, and the Clinical AIDS Study Group, 1989, "Detection of HIV-2 infection and ratio to HIV-1 among hopsitalized patients in Rio de Janiero, Brazil" *Proceedings* V International Conference on AIDS, Montreal, 4-9 June, abstract T.G.P.25

Smallman-Raynor M R, Cliff A D, 1990a, "Acquired immune deficiency syndrome (AIDS): literature, geographical origins and global patterns" *Progress in Human Geography* forthcoming

Smallman-Raynor M R, Cliff A D, 1990b, "The simian origin hypothesis and dispersal of human immunodeficiency viruses in Africa: a geographical perspective", submitted to *Reviews of Infectious Diseases* details from authors on request

Smith T F, Srinivasan A, Schoechetma G, Marcus M, Myers G, 1988, "The phylogenetic history of immunodeficiency viruses" *Nature* **339** 573–575

Somsé P, Georges A J, Siopathis R M, Vohito J A, Bouquety J C, Vohito M D, 1989, "Les aspects epidemiologiques des affections liees aux VIH1 et 3 en Republic Centrafricaine" *Proceedings* V International Conference on AIDS, Montreal, 4–9 June, abstract W.G.O.28

Soriano V, Tor J, Ribera A, Fernandez J L, Muga R, Fox M, 1989a, "Retrovirus infection (HIV-1, HIV-2, HTLV-1) in asymptomatic West Africans living in Spain" *Proceedings* V International Conference on AIDS, Montreal, 4–9 June, abstract A.556

Soriano V, Tor J, Ribera A, Muga R, Clotet B, Martin J, 1989b, "HIV-2 in drug users of Spain" *Proceedings* V International Conference on AIDS, Montreal, 4–9 June, abstract M.A.P.81

Sow A, Coll Awa M, Fayendao M A, Diouf G, Feller-Dansokho E, Diop B M, 1989, "Aspects cliniques HIV1 et HIV2 et classification de Bangui" *Proceedings* V International Conference on AIDS, Montreal, 4–9 June, abstract M.B.P.195

Teas J, 1983, "Could AIDS agent be a new variant of African swine fever virus" *Lancet* **1** 923

Tedder R S, O'Connor T, Hughes A, N'jie H, Corrah T, Whittle H, 1988, "Envelope cross-reactivity in Western blot for HIV-1 and HIV-2 may not indicate dual infection" *Lancet* **ii** 927–930

Toh H, Miyata T, 1985, "Is the AIDS virus a recombinant?" *Nature* **316** 21–22

Torres Pereira N, Louro Rodrigues J M, 1988, "A prevalência da infecçâo por virus HIV na experiência do serviço de imunohemoterapia dos hositais civis de Lisboa" *Arquivos do Instituto Bacteriológico Câmara Pestana* **4** 47–52

Traore I, Pichard E, Traore M L, 1988, "Aspects radiologiques de l'atteinte des membres au cours de la maladi de Kaposi: a propos de 4 case" *Médecine d'Afrique Noire* **35** 948–949

Tricoire J, Robert A, Puel J, Brun-Vézinet F, Gayet C, Régnier C, 1989, "Contamination d'un jeune hemophile par le virus VIH 2" *Proceedings* V International Conference on AIDS, Montreal, 4–9 June, abstract Th.B.P.21

Tumani Corrah E A A, Wilkins A, Gaye F, Whittle H, Greenwood B, 1989, "Clinical characterization of HIV-2 disease in West Africa" *Proceedings* V International Conference on AIDS, Montreal, 4–9 June, abstract T.B.P.362

Van de Perre P, Rouvroy D, Lepage P, Bogaerts J, Kestelyn P, Kayihigi J, Hekker A C, Butzlier J P, Clumeck N, 1984, "Acquired immunodeficiency syndrome in Rwanda" *Lancet* **ii** 62–65

Vanderborght B, de Leys R J, Nijs P, Van de Groen G, Merregaert J, Prinsen H, van Heuverswyn H, 1988, "Isolation of human immunodeficiency virus type 2 from a homosexual man in Belgium" *European Journal of Clinical Microbiology and Infectious Diseases* **7** 816–818

Varnier O E, Lillo F B, Schito G C, Lazzarin A, Kanki P J, 1988, "Parallel Western blot analysis for HIV-1 and HIV-2 antibodies: absence of HIV-2 infection in Italian subjects at risk for AIDS" *AIDS* **2** 215–217

Verdier M, Sangaré A, Sassou-Guesseau E, Gaye A, Al-Qubati G, Denis F, 1989, "Etude comparee des prevalences HIV-1, HIV-2 et HTLV-1 chez les lepreux de 4 pays: Cote d'Ivoire, Congo, Senegal, Yemen" *Proceedings* V International Conference on AIDS, Montreal, 4–9 June, abstract T.B.O.9

Veronesi R, Mazza C C, Ferreira M O S, Lourenço M H, 1987, "HIV-2 in Brazil" *Lancet* **ii** 402

Victorino R, Teles L C, Ferreira M O, Guerreiro O, Lourenço M H, 1989, "Analysis of a screening program for HIV1 and HIV2 infection in women of reproductive age" *Proceedings* V International Conference on AIDS, Montreal, 4-9 June, abstract A.512

Vilmer E, Rouzioux C, Vézinet-Brun F, Fischer A, Chermann J C, Barré-Sinoussi F, Gazengel C, Dauguet C, Manigne P, Griscelli C, 1984, "Isolation of new lymphotropic retroviruses from two siblings with haemophilia B, one with AIDS" *Lancet* i 753-757

Vittecoq D, Ferchal F, Chamaret S, Benbunan M, Gerber M, Hirsch A, Montagnier L, 1987, "Routes of HIV-2 transmission in Western Europe" *Lancet* i 1150-1151

Weiss S H, Lombardo J, Michaels J, Sharer L R, Tyyarah M, Leonard J, Mongia A, Kloser P, Sathe S, Kapila R, Williams N M, Altman R, French J, Parkin W E, 1988, "AIDS due to HIV-2 infection—New Jersey" *Journal of the American Medical Association* **259** 969-970

Werner A, Staszewski S, Helm E B, Stille W, Weber K, Kurth R, 1987, "HIV-2 (West Germany, 1984)" *Lancet* i 868-869

WHO, 1988, "Acquired Immunodeficiency Syndrome (AIDS)—data as at 31 December 1987", World Health Organization *Weekly Epidemiological Record* **63** 14-15

WHO, 1989, "Acquired immunodeficiency syndrome (AIDS)—data as at 30 June 1989" World Health Organization *Weekly Epidemiological* **64** 205-206

Williams E, Hearst N, Udofia O, 1989, "Sexual practices and HIV infection of female prostitutes in Nigeria" *Proceedings* V International Conference on AIDS, Montreal, 4-9 June, abstract W.G.O.24

Winkler E, Holten I, Meyer A, Rehle T, Garin D, Mefane C, Parry J V, Schmitz H, 1989, "Seroepidemiology of human retroviruses in Gabon" *AIDS* 3 106-107

Wolfheim J H, 1983 *Primates of the World: Distribution, Abundance, and Conservation* (University of Washington Press, Seattle, WA)

Yala F, Biendo M, Madzouka J, Copin N, Carne B, 1989, "Absence actuelle de HIV-2 a Brazzaville (Congo)" *Proceedings* V International Conference on AIDS, Montreal, 4-9 June, abstract A.568

Yokoyama S, Chung L, Gojobori T, 1988, "Molecular evolution of the human immunodeficiency and related viruses" *Molecular Biology and Evolution* **5** 237-251

Zewdie D, Woody J, Ayhumie S, Constantine B, Gebrehiwot B, Messele T, Gizaw G, 1989, "Human immunodeficiency virus type 2 (HIV-2) screening of a high risk population in Addis Ababa, Ethiopia" *Proceedings* V International Conference on AIDS, Montreal, 4-9 June, abstract M.A.P.79

APPENDIX 1
A1 Human immunodeficiency virus type 2
A1.1 Isolation of HIV-1

The first isolation of the causative agent of AIDS in man was made in France by Barré-Sinoussi et al (1983) who named the virus 'LAV' (lymphadenopathy-associated retrovirus). Gallo et al (1984) made the second isolation in the USA and termed the virus 'HTLV-III (human T-lymphotropic virus type III). Because of this duplication and of the suggestion that Gallo had, in fact, reisolated the same virus as the French group, the convention was to term the virus LAV/HTLV-III or HTLV-III/LAV. The nomenclature was confused further by the terminology applied to subsequent isolations of the virus in the same year in the USA: 'ARV' (AIDS-associated retrovirus; see Levy et al, 1984) and 'IDAV' (immuno-deficiency-associated virus; see Vilmer et al, 1984). Eventually, the International Committee on Taxonomy of Viruses resolved matters by proposing the term 'human immunodeficiency virus' (HIV) to cover all strains of the causative virus of AIDS in man (Coffin et al, 1986). LAV /HTLV-III was reclassified as HIV-1.

A1.2 Isolation of HIV-2

The first indication of the existence of another human immunodeficiency virus, related to HIV-1, came with the isolation in 1986 of a possible fourth human retrovirus, 'HTLV-IV' (human T-lymphotropic virus type IV), by Kanki et al (1986) from West African prostitutes. These isolates were later shown to be laboratory contaminations of a genuine new strain of HIV by a simian immunodeficiency virus isolated from captive rhesus monkeys (*Macaca mulatta*) (Kestler et al, 1988; Mulder et al, 1988). This genuine second strain of HIV, originally termed 'LAV-II' (lymphadenopathy-associated retrovirus type II) but later renamed HIV-2, was definitively isolated in 1986 by researchers at the Pasteur Institute in France from AIDS patients originating from the former Portuguese West African colonies of Guinea-Bissau and Cape Verde (Clavel et al, 1986). Subsequent reisolations of the virus were made in 1987 (Brun-Vézinet et al, 1987).

A1.3 Relationship of HIV-1 and HIV-2

HIV (covering both strains) is a retrovirus. A retrovirus is a virus of higher organisms whose genome is RNA, but which can insert a DNA copy of its genome into the host's chromosome. The virus thus becomes a permanent part of the infected person's own cells. Genomic sequencing has indicated that HIV is more closely related to mammalian viruses of the Lentivirus subfamily of retroviruses than to the Oncovirus subfamily to which human T-lymphotropic virus types I and II (HTLV-I and II), the 'first human retroviruses', belong (Gonda et al, 1986).

HIV-1 and HIV-2 are related, but genetically distinct, viruses sharing 30–60% amino acid sequence homology between their genes (Chakrabarti et al, 1987; Fukasawa et al, 1988). In terms of genomic organisation,

HIV-1 contains an open reading frame, *vpu*, absent from HIV-2, and HIV-2 contains an open reading frame, *vpx*, absent from HIV-1 (Clavel, 1987; Essex and Kanki, 1988; Peterlin and Luciw, 1988). The function of these genes remains uncertain, although, as discussed below (subsection A1.5), they may play a part in the reproductive and pathogenic capabilities of the two viruses (Essex and Kanki, 1988).

A1.4 Transmission corridors of HIV-2

Transmission corridors for HIV-2 appear to parallel those for HIV-1 (*Lancet*, 1988); infection by homosexual and heterosexual contact, contaminated blood products, and from mother to child have all been reported (Biesert et al, 1988; Brücker et al, 1987; Ouattara et al, 1988; Tumani Corrah et al, 1989). However, decreased efficiency for both heterosexual transmission (Kanki et al, 1989; Poulsen et al, 1989b) and perinatal transmission (Andreasson et al, 1989; Kvinesdal et al, 1989; Poulsen et al, 1989a) of HIV-2 relative to HIV-1 has been proposed.

A1.5 Incubation period and pathogenic potential of HIV-2

Estimates of the mean incubation period (that is, the time-lag between primary infection and development of AIDS) for HIV-1 infection range from 4 to 15 years (Lui et al, 1986; 1988; Medley et al, 1987; Rees, 1987), but the incubation period for HIV-2 infection is even more uncertain. The virus has been observed for only a short length of time and there is a lack of information regarding the time of exposure of individuals to it. Reports of HIV-2-infected Europeans believed to have been exposed to the virus in West Africa, suggest extraordinarily long incubation periods of 19 years or more for this strain (Ancelle et al, 1987; Dufoort et al, 1988).

Initial isolations of HIV-2 were made from individuals in West Africa who displayed AIDS or ARC (AIDS-related complex) (Brun-Vézinet et al, 1987; Clavel et al, 1986). Subsequently, AIDS cases associated with HIV-2 have been reported from 3 continents (Ayres et al, 1989; Le Guenno et al, 1987a; Neumann et al, 1989b; Oelman et al, 1989). In a number of studies, immunological perturbations during stages of HIV-2 infection paralleling those in the progression to HIV-1-associated AIDS have been observed (Le Guenno and Sarthou, 1989; Lisse et al, 1989); isolations of HIV-2 strains presenting purely as neurological disorders have also been made (Evans et al, 1988a; Kong et al, 1988). Although this is evidence for the pathogenic capability of HIV-2, the findings are not sufficient in themselves to define causality, and cohort studies suggest that HIV-2 has a lower pathogenic capability than HIV-1 (Romieu et al, 1989).

The first piece of evidence for low pathogenic potential comes from follow-up studies of disease development in initially asymptomatic HIV-2 seropositive cohorts in West Africa. For example, Marlink et al (1989) report on a 27-month follow-up study of 60 initially asympomatic HIV-2 seropositive female prostitutes in Senegal. If HIV-2 had the same pathogenic capability as HIV-1 (as determined by studies of similar cohorts in Zaire) 13 cases of ARC and 11 cases of AIDS would have been expected in the Senegalese cohort over the study period. Yet Marlink and co-workers have failed to detect any significant development of disease.

The second piece of evidence for low pathogenic potential comes from the age-specific distribution of HIV-2 infection in cohorts studied in West Africa. Several reports detail a rising prevalence of HIV-2 infection with age. This evidence contrasts with the typical peak prevalence of HIV-1 in the 20–30 years age-group (Essex and Kanki, 1988; Kanki et al, 1987; 1989; Pepin et al, 1989; Poulsen et al, 1989b). In figure A1 this unusual epidemiological contrast is shown by comparing the age-specific and sex-specific incidence of AIDS cases associated with HIV-1, reported in Uganda (Central Africa), with age-specific and sex-specific HIV-2 seroprevalence data from a study of randomly selected individuals from Bissau City, Guinea-Bissau (West Africa). Peak prevalence of

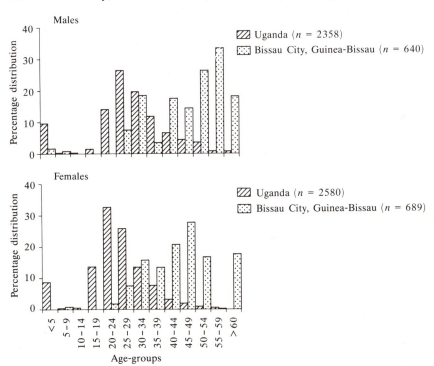

Figure A1. Age-specific distribution of reported AIDS cases associated with HIV-1 in males and females in Uganda, Central Africa, to July 1988 and age-specific distribution of HIV-2 infection prevalence in randomly selected males and females in Bissau City, Guinea-Bissau, West Africa, in 1987. Sources: drawn from Berkley et al, 1989; Poulsen et al, 1989b.

HIV-1-associated AIDS (as a surrogate for the age-specific distribution
of HIV-1 infection) occurs in the 20–34 years age-groups, whereas peak
prevalence of HIV-2 infection occurs in the over-45 age-group. Such
findings suggest that HIV-2 is not removing individuals from the population
through HIV-related disease in the same way as HIV-1 (Essex and Kanki,
1988; Kanki et al, 1987; 1989).

The conflicting evidence regarding the disease-causing potential of
HIV-2 can be reconciled by the possible existence of a mixture of
pathogenic and nonpathogenic strains in the population, and it is becoming
increasingly evident that variability in HIV-2 strain is at least as great as
that of HIV-1 (Rübsamen-Waigmann et al, 1989). Differential disease
development may also be arising because of the recent import of HIV-2
into some countries (Clavel et al, 1987). Whatever the long-term
pathogenic potential of HIV-2, observations in West Africa of AIDS
cases associated with HIV-2 suggest that the clinical spectrum of disease
does not differ significantly from that associated with HIV-1 (Gody et al,
1988; Odehouri et al, 1989; Sow et al, 1989; Tumani Corrah et al, 1989).

A1.6 Antigenic cross-reactivity and the diagnosis of HIV-2 infection
Few 'pedigree' isolations of HIV-2 have been made, and, as a result, it
has not been possible to evaluate the accuracy of diagnostic tests for the
virus (*Lancet*, 1988). The problem of antigenic cross-reactivity in the
determination of HIV status is particularly acute: serological tests for HIV-2
infection may react as a result of the presence of antibodies to HIV-1
even in confirmatory testing procedures. As a result, dual HIV-1/HIV-2
infection may be falsely suspected when only HIV-1 infection exists
(Böttiger et al, 1988; Buttò et al, 1988; Schmidt et al, 1989; Tedder
et al, 1988). It is also apparent that there are geographical variations in
the degree of viral cross-reactivity. This may be evidence of variation in
HIV strain, the existence of genuine new HIVs or variations in immune
response (Simon et al, 1989a). Essex (1989) suggests, on the strength of
the cross-reactivity problem, that dual infection is very rare and that
such reports must be treated with caution. However, definitive cases of
dual infection have been identified (Evans et al, 1988b; Rouzioux et al,
1989).

APPENDIX 2
A2 Simian immunodeficiency viruses and the origins of HIV
A2.1 Origin hypotheses

Many hypotheses have been proposed for the origin of HIV. Early suggestions were that HIV may have (1) evolved from viruses of pigs (African swine fever virus; see Teas, 1983) or chickens (Rous sarcoma virus; see Moore and Le Baron, 1986); (2) evolved from bovine visna virus (Grote, 1988); (3) resulted from genetic manipulation in Western laboratories (Modrow et al, 1987; Sabatier, 1988); or (4) from molecular recombination in vivo (McClure and Schulz, 1989; Toh and Miyata, 1985). Retrospective serological analysis has, however, indicated that HIV was circulating in Africa in the 1960s or before, and this continent has become the focus of studies seeking to establish the hearth of the virus. We have given an overview of the evidence in another paper (Smallman-Raynor and Cliff, 1990a).

A2.2 Origins of HIV-2

The most widely held view is that HIV developed from related immunodeficiency viruses found in nonhuman African primates. Recent analysis has suggested that a simian immunodeficiency virus, called SIVman, from the African sooty mangabey (*Cercocebus atys*) may be the direct progenitor of HIV-2 (Hirsch et al, 1989; Li et al, 1989). The earliest isolations of SIVman were made in 1986 from captive monkeys in the USA (Fultz et al, 1986; Lowenstine et al, 1986; Murphey-Corb et al, 1986), and retrospective serological analysis has shown evidence of infection in US cohorts as early as 1968 (Hirsch et al, 1989). The first reports of possible wild infection with SIVman came in 1988 (Montagnier, 1988)—reports that were confirmed in 1989 (Hirsch et al, 1989). SIVman is very closely related in nucleotide sequence homology terms both to HIV-2 and to SIVmac, a simian immunodeficiency virus of the Asian rhesus monkey, *Macaca mulata*. The three viruses form a major immuno-deficiency virus subgrouping (Hirsch et al, 1989; Li et al, 1989), and the natural range of the sooty mangabey coincides directly with the West African area of known HIV-2 endemicity (see figure 4). It is thus hypothesised by Hirsch et al (1989) that there have been two independent emergences of HIV: HIV-2 in West Africa due to cross-species transmission of SIVman; and HIV-1 in Central Africa due to cross-species transmission of a simian immunodeficiency virus of the African green monkey, SIVagm, or of a related SIV from other Central African monkey species (Hirsch et al, 1989).

APPENDIX 3
A3 Epidemiology of HIV-2
A3.1 Africa
A3.1.1 *Transmission routes*
The whole of tropical Africa, covering areas of endemic infection with
both HIV-1 and HIV-2, is classified by the World Health Organization
as a region displaying pattern II AIDS/HIV infection (Mann et al, 1988;
Piot et al, 1988). Under this classification, the dominant routes of
transmission are heterosexual contact, vertical transmission from mother
to child, and blood or blood-product receipt. These characteristics
contrast markedly with the pattern I regions of the developed West.
Pattern I regions are characterised by homosexual and intravenous-drug-
abuser routes of infection, and these corridors are believed to be rare
or absent in pattern II areas (Mann et al, 1988; Piot et al, 1988).

There is some doubt regarding the efficiency of HIV-2 transmission
heterosexually relative to that of HIV-1 (Kanki et al, 1989; Poulsen
et al, 1989b). However, the centrality of heterosexual activity in the
HIV-2 epidemic is supported by the extraordinarily high rates of infection
in female prostitutes and, to a lesser extent, in pregnant women and
heterosexual STD (sexually transmitted disease) patients. See the discussion
of table A1, below. The dominance of the heterosexual transmission
route is further confirmed by the parity of the male : female ratio in
HIV-2 AIDS cases and infection in many West African countries (Oelman
et al, 1989; Poulsen et al, 1989b).

There is also doubt regarding the efficiency of perinatal HIV-2
transmission relative to that of HIV-1 (Andreasson et al, 1989; Kvinesdal
et al, 1989; Poulsen et al, 1989a; Tumani Corrah et al, 1989).

Among blood donors, HIV-2 prevalence in West Africa varies. Rates
range from 0.23% in Guinea (Foucault-Fretz et al, 1989) to 17.6% in
Guinea-Bissau (Nauclér et al, 1989) where definitive reports of transmission
through blood receipt have been made (Couroucé, 1987; Couroucé
et al, 1988; Ouattara et al, 1988). There is, additionally, some evidence
from Mozambique of HIV-2 transmission during scarification rituals
(de la Cruz, personal communication, see footnote 4).

A3.1.2 *Epidemiology of HIV-2 infection*
The degree of penetration of HIV-2 into various risk and nonrisk
populations in the nations of West and South Central Africa is shown in
table A1. Findings from general practice are used as controls. As with
the epidemiology of HIV-1 in Central Africa, female prostitutes display the
greatest rates of infection, although high rates of infection are also
found in cohorts of the general population of some countries. In this
part of the continent, the geography of HIV-2 infection is complex and
varies at all geographical scales. At the international level, highest rates
of infection in risk and nonrisk cohorts are recorded in Guinea-Bissau

and surrounding regions. That Guinea-Bissau is the focus of the HIV-2 epidemic is suggested by the fact that HIV-2 prevalence among female prostitutes in neighbouring Senegal ranges from 1.5% in Saint Louis on the northern border with Mauritania, to 46% in Ziguinchor on the southern Senegalese border with Guinea-Bissau (M'Boup et al, 1989). In Guinea-Bissau itself, prevalence among groups varies regionally and locally. For example, Andreasson et al (1989) note among pregnant women in Guinea-Bissau a prevalence of HIV-2 infection ranging from 3.6% in Catio in the south of the country close to the Guinea border, to 7% in Bissau City. At the local scale, HIV-2 infection among pregnant women ranges from 3.5% to 12.3% in different parts of Bissau City (Andreasson et al, 1989).

In the South Central African states, in Angola, prevalence rates for HIV-2 as high as 16% for blood donors, 6.8% for pregnant women, and 10.5% in STD patients have been recorded in the towns in the northeast of the country (Matos-Almeida et al, 1989). In Mozambique, extensive serological analyses conducted in major towns and cities throughout the country have revealed prevalences in the general population of 1.69% in males and 1.41% in females, with estimates of upwards of 16 500 HIV-2 infections in these urban areas (de la Cruz et al, 1989).

Table A1. Results of serological screening for HIV-2 infection in West and South Central Africa. Source: Romieu et al, 1989 (exceptions indicated by footnotes).

Country	HIV-2 positive per number tested (%)			
	general practice	heterosexual STD patients	pregnant women	female prostitutes
West Africa				
Benin	0.0	nd	0.0	3.7
Burkina Faso	0.0	15.6	1.7	20.4
Cape Verde	11.4	nd	nd	nd
Gambia	1.6	5.0	nd	3.0[a]
Ghana[b]	nd	nd	nd	7.3
Guinea	0.0	nd	1.7	nd
Guinea-Bissau	8.3	6.0	8.5	33.3
Ivory Coast	0.9	nd	3.3	20.0
Mali	nd	nd	3.0	34.0
Senegal	0.6	1.9	4.2	11.0
Sierra Leone[c]	nd	1.8	nd	nd
South Central Africa				
Angola[d]	nd	10.5	nd	nd
Mozambique[e]	1.6	nd	nd	nd

nd no data.
[a] Mabey et al, 1988. [b] Fleming, 1988. [c] Kosia et al, 1989. [d] Matos-Almeida et al, 1989. [e] de la Cruz et al, 1989.

In table A2 the occurrence of HIV-1 and HIV-2 infection in some West African states and in Angola/Mozambique is compared. Considerable variability is evident. In Mozambique and Ivory Coast, for example, both virus strains appear to have penetrated equally, although in Senegal HIV-2 is the dominant virus. The majority of AIDS cases reported in many West and South Central African nations are associated with HIV-1 rather than HIV-2 infection (de la Cruz et al, 1989; Gody et al, 1988), although AIDS cases associated with HIV-2 have been recorded in most countries of endemic HIV-2 infection (de la Cruz et al, 1989; Gody et al, 1988; Le Guenno et al, 1987a; 1987b; Matos-Almeida et al, 1989; Nauclér et al, 1989; Oelman et al, 1989; Traore et al, 1988).

Table A2. Comparative prevalences of HIV-1 and HIV-2 infection in various groups from West and South Central Africa.

Country	Group	Date	Prevalance (%)	
			HIV-1	HIV-2
Angola[a]	STD patients	1987	11.0	10.5
	Blood donors	1987	8.0	16.0
Burkina Faso[b]	Prostitutes	1986	8.8	14.6
Ghana[c]	Prostitutes	1986–87	25.2	7.3
Guinea[d]	Blood donors	1987–88	0.2	0.2
Ivory Coast[e]	Healthy urban	1987–88	1.5	1.5
Mozambique[f]	Healthy urban	1987–88	1.1	1.2
Senegal[g]	Prostitutes	1987	1.2	9.9
Sierra Leone[h]	STD patients	1988	2.1	1.8

[a] Matos-Almeida et al, 1989. [b] Sangaré et al, 1989. [c] Fleming, 1988.
[d] Foucault-Fretz et al, 1989. [e] Gody et al, 1988. [f] de la Cruz et al, 1989.
[g] Kanki et al, 1989. [h] Kosia et al, 1989.

A3.2 Europe

A3.2.1 *HIV-2 infections*

Study of 40 sources relating to the occurrence of HIV-2 in Europe to June 1989 reveals a total of 205 unique HIV-2 infections (including possible repeat reports). In table A3, we show the country and the likely source (internal or external to the continent) of infection by using the data which form the basis of the spread diagram, figure 9. An additional 160 dual HIV-1/HIV-2 infections detected in Europe, probably resulting from the antigenic cross-reactivity problem described in appendix 1, are shown in table A4.

Table A3. Unique HIV-2 infections detected in Europe.

Country	Number HIV-2 positive	Source of infection external	Source of infection internal	No data or poor data
Belgium[a, b]	3	2		1
FRG[c]	25	16		9
Finland[d]	1	1		
France[a, e, f]	37	24	4 + (8?)	1
Greece[g]	1			1
Italy[h]	6	2	4	
Luxembourg[e]	1	1		
Norway[i]	1			1
Portugal[j]	117	72	9	36
Spain[k]	3	3		
USSR[l]	7	6	1	
United Kingdom[m]	3	2		1
Total	205	129	26	50

Note: These figures may include some repeat reports which cannot be disentangled from the published data.
[a] Vittecoq et al, 1987. [b] Vanderborght et al, 1988. [c] Biesert et al, 1988; Kroegel et al, 1987; Werner et al, 1987. [d] Leinikki et al, 1989. [e] Simon et al, 1989b. [f] Ancelle et al, 1987; Brücker et al, 1987; Couroucé, 1987; Couroucé et al, 1988; Dufoort et al, 1988; Saimot et al, 1987. [g] Fountouli et al, 1989. [h] Pintus et al, 1989; Scasso et al, 1988. [i] Kingman, 1987. [j] Ayres et al, 1989; Botas et al, 1989; Bryceson et al, 1988; Cardoso et al, 1989; Saal et al, 1987; Victorino et al, 1989. [k] Soriano et al, 1989a. [l] Pokrovskii et al, 1988. [m] BHTD, 1988; Heath et al, 1988; Loveday et al, 1989.

Table A4. Dual HIV-1/HIV-2 infections detected in Europe.

Country	Number HIV-1/HIV-2 positive
France[a]	10
Greece[b]	9
Italy[c]	132
Spain[d]	9
Total	160

[a] Couroucé et al, 1988; Rey et al, 1987; Rouzioux et al, 1989. [b] Georgoulias et al, 1988. [c] Cadeo et al, 1989; Ferroni et al, 1987; Martegani et al, 1988; Pintus et al, 1989; Scasso et al, 1988. [d] Soriano et al, 1989b.

APPENDIX 4
A4 Sources of selected figures
A4.1 Sources of figure 3 (countries for which HIV-2 screening has been reported)

Agius et al, 1989
Ancelle et al, 1987
Ayanian et al, 1989
Ayres et al, 1989
Bayliss et al, 1988
BHTD, 1988
Biesert et al, 1988
Botas et al, 1989
Böttiger et al, 1988
Bouzas et al, 1989
Brücker et al, 1987
Bryceson et al, 1988
Cadeo et al, 1989
Cardoso et al, 1989
Chevallier et al, 1989
Constantine et al, 1989
Contreras et al, 1989
Cortes et al, 1989a
Cour et al, 1989
Couroucé, 1987
Couroucé et al, 1988
De Cock et al, 1989
de la Cruz[6]
de la Cruz et al, 1989
Denis et al, 1987
Dufoort et al, 1988
Essien and Saliu, 1989
Ferroni et al, 1987
Fleming, 1988
Foucault-Fretz et al, 1989
Fountouli et al, 1989
Georges et al, 1988
Georgoulias et al, 1988
Gody et al, 1988
Gresenguet et al, 1988
Heath et al, 1988
Horsburgh and Holmberg, 1988
Ishikawa et al, 1988
Kanki et al, 1987; 1989
Kaptue et al, 1989

Kawamura et al, 1989
Kingman, 1987
Kosia et al, 1989
Kroegel et al, 1987
Lecatsas et al, 1989
Leinikki et al, 1989
Lourenço et al, 1989
Loveday et al, 1989
Lyons et al, 1988a; 1988b; 1989
Mabey et al, 1988
Malkin et al, 1989
Mannuci et al, 1989
Martegani et al, 1988
Matos-Almeida et al, 1989
M'Boup et al, 1989
Mertens et al, 1989
Mintz et al, 1988
Mohammed et al, 1989
Nakamura et al, 1987
Nauclér et al, 1989
Neumann et al, 1988; 1989a; 1989b
Oelman et al, 1989
Ouattara et al, 1988; 1989
Ousséini et al, 1989
Palha de Sousa et al, 1989
Pepin et al, 1989
Pintus et al, 1989
Pokrovskii et al, 1988
Poulsen et al, 1989b
Rey et al, 1986; 1987
Ricard et al, 1989
Romieu et al, 1989
Rouzioux et al, 1989
Rwandan HIVSG, 1989
Saal et al, 1987
Saimot et al, 1987
Sangaré et al, 1989
Santos-Ferreira et al, 1989
Scasso et al, 1988

[6] Personal communication, see footnote 5, page 151.

Shanmugasundararaj et al, 1988
Simon et al, 1989a
Sion et al, 1989
Somsé et al, 1989
Soriano et al, 1989a; 1989b
Torres Pereira and Louro
    Rodrigues, 1988
Traore et al, 1988
Tricoire et al, 1989
Vanderborght et al, 1988
Varnier et al, 1988

Verdier et al, 1989
Veronesi et al, 1987
Victorino et al, 1989
Vittecoq et al, 1987
Weiss et al, 1988
Werner et al, 1987
Williams et al, 1989
Winkler et al, 1989
Yala et al, 1989
Zewdie et al, 1989

A4.2 Sources of figure 5(a) (countries reporting unique HIV-2 infection within their borders) and 5(b) (countries reporting only dual HIV-1/HIV-2 within their borders)

(a)

Ancelle et al, 1987
Ayres et al, 1989
BHTD, 1988
Biesert et al, 1988
Botas et al, 1989
Böttiger et al, 1988
Brücker et al, 1987
Bryceson et al, 1988
Cardoso et al, 1989
Clavel et al, 1987
Couroucé, 1987
Couroucé et al, 1988
De Cock et al, 1989
de la Cruz[7]
de la Cruz et al, 1989
Denis et al, 1987
Dufoort et al, 1988
Essien and Saliu, 1989
Fleming, 1988
Foucault-Fretz et al, 1989
Fountouli et al, 1989
Georges et al, 1988
Gody et al, 1988
Heath et al, 1988
Ishikawa et al, 1988
Kanki et al, 1989
Kawamura et al, 1989
Kingman, 1987
Kosia et al, 1989

Kroegel et al, 1987
Leinikki et al, 1989
Lourenço et al, 1989
Loveday et al, 1989
Lyons et al, 1988b; 1989
Mabey et al, 1988
Malkin et al, 1989
Matos-Almeida et al, 1989
M'Boup et al, 1989
Mohammed et al, 1989
Nauclér et al, 1989
Neumann et al, 1988; 1989a;
    1989b
Oelman et al, 1989
Ouattara et al, 1988; 1989
Ousséini et al, 1989
Palha de Sousa et al, 1989
Pepin et al, 1989
Pintus et al, 1989
Pokrovskii et al, 1988
Poulsen et al, 1989b
Ricard et al, 1989
Romieu et al, 1989
Rwandan HIVSG, 1989
Saal et al, 1987
Saimot et al, 1987
Sangaré et al, 1989
Santos-Ferreira et al, 1989
Scasso et al, 1988

[7] Personal communication, see footnote 5, page 151.

Simon et al, 1989a
Sion et al, 1989
Somsé et al, 1989
Soriano et al, 1989a
Torres Pereira and Louro
  Rodrigues, 1988
Traore et al, 1988
Tricoire et al, 1989
Veronesi et al, 1987
Victorino et al, 1989
Vittecoq et al, 1987
Weiss et al, 1988
Werner et al, 1987
Williams et al, 1989
Winkler et al, 1989

(b)
Constantine et al, 1989
Kaptue et al, 1989
Lyons et al, 1988a
Shanmugasundararaj et al, 1988
Zewdie et al, 1989

A4.3 Sources of figure 8 (the diffusion of HIV-2 within Africa)

Bigot et al, 1987 (1)
Böttiger et al, 1988 (2)
Clavel et al, 1987 (3)
de la Cruz[8] (4)
Denis et al, 1987 (5)
Georges et al, 1988 (6)
Ishikawa et al, 1988 (7)
Kaptue et al, 1989 (8)
Konotey-Ahulu, 1989 (9)

Lyons et al, 1988a (10); 1989 (11)
Mabey et al, 1988 (12)
Neequaye et al, 1986 (13);
  1988 (14)
Ouattara et al, 1986 (15)
Pepin et al, 1989 (16)
Rwandan HIVSG, 1989 (17)
Schoub et al, 1988 (18)
Winkler et al, 1989 (19)

Numbers in brackets refer to the numbers on the figure.

A4.4 Sources of figure 9 (the diffusion of HIV-2 into Europe)

Ancelle et al, 1987 (1)
Ayres et al, 1989 (2)
BHTD, 1988 (6)
Biesert et al, 1988 (3)
Botas et al, 1989 (4)
Bryceson et al, 1988 (5)
Cardoso et al, 1989 (7)
Couroucé, 1987 (8)
Couroucé et al, 1988 (9)
Dufoort et al, 1988 (10)
Heath et al, 1988 (11)
Kroegel et al, 1987 (12)

Leinikki et al, 1989 (13)
Pintus et al, 1989 (14)
Pokrovskii et al, 1988 (15)
Saal et al, 1987 (16)
Saimot et al, 1987 (17)
Scasso et al, 1988 (18)
Simon et al, 1989a (19)
Soriano et al, 1989a (20)
Victorino et al, 1989 (21)
Vittecoq et al, 1987 (22)
Werner et al, 1987 (23)

Numbers in brackets refer to numbers in the figure.

[8] Personal communication, see footnote 5, page 151.

Reflections on the AIDS Distribution Pattern in the United States of America

A K DUTT, D MILLER
University of Akron, OH
H M DUTTA
Kent State University, OH

1 Introduction

In the USA the human immunodeficiency virus (HIV) was originally a disease agent found to be limited primarily to the homosexual community. In 1990, it is still a disease carried mainly by homosexuals, but is spreading fast among intravenous (IV) drug abusers. The specific origin of the virus is uncertain, but it is believed to have been brought into the USA from countries where the chief method of transmission is through heterosexual contact. In a previous paper, I (Dutt) and others pointed out that AIDS originated in Africa (Dutt et al, 1987) and a year later Shannon and Pyle prepared a 'global' AIDS diffusion map showing how the disease spread from a Central African source (Shannon and Pyle, 1989). Later studies of AIDS have confirmed that there are now two HIV viruses—HIV-1 and HIV-2—the first one concentrated in Central Africa and the second one in West Africa in Cape Verde, Guinea, and Senegal (Brooke, 1989). It has also been suggested that the Ivory Coast is the meeting ground of the two viruses (Brooke, 1989). Though HIV-2 has entered Europe, its entrance into the USA is very limited, though eventually might spread all over the world. Therefore, another diffusion map based on the spread of HIV-2 is needed (see Smallman-Raynor and Cliff, this volume) to supplement the work by Shannon and Pyle (1989).

Fully developed AIDS cases have been reported in 117781 people in the USA up to 31 December 1989, and 59.8% of the adults and adolescents diagnosed as AIDS patients died, according to figures from a joint survey by the US Department of Health and Education and the US Centers for Disease Control (CDC) (USDHE/CDC, 1990). In a new revised calculation, CDC also affirms that another 800000 to 1300000 people are already infected with HIV (Palca, 1989). It should be noted here that there is a difference between a person being tested as positive with HIV and the evidence of the onslaught of the opportunistic diseases that are the result of immunodeficiency known as AIDS, according to the standards established by the CDC in Atlanta, GA (Thomas, 1986). It is quite possible that everyone infected with the virus will eventually die from the disease, unless a curative medicine is discovered. In this paper, the statistical analysis will be based on fully developed AIDS cases in the USA.

This paper will address the development and increase of new types of patient, and the progress of the epidemic will also be reported and charted.

These new proportions should be taken into consideration when education programs are designed and implemented and also when health departments develop projections and establish plans for treatment and facilities, and programs for the future. The magnitude of these trends must be taken seriously because, as the former US Surgeon General, C Everett Koop, advises, "AIDS is virtually 100% fatal" (Koop, 1989, page 113).

In this paper, we will give an overview, with statistics obtained from CDC, of the regional and national distribution both of the established types of patient and of the new types of patient. The percentages are examined by age, gender, and race to help bring the trends into focus. Moreover, this study is a follow-up report of the 1987 study made by myself and others (Dutt et al, 1987). In this paper we will also address the spread of AIDS: in particular the overall shifting of regional patterns that have varied greatly since 1981.

In the USA, the concentration of AIDS cases was originally focused in three large metropolitan areas, New York City, San Francisco, and Los Angeles. Over time, the disease has begun to disburse from these three primary large Metropolitan Statistical Areas (MSAs) to the Northeast, West, and South, and thence throughout the rest of the USA.

Figures now reflect the concentration in the large MSAs centered around the New York/New Jersey/Connecticut area in the Northeast and in the San Francisco/Los Angeles area in the West. New York and New Jersey both claim to have the highest incidence of AIDS (Joseph, 1988). In addition, Florida and Washington DC also have very high rates of incidence of AIDS. In 1989, 7 cities reported 40 and above cases of AIDS per year per 100000 people: San Francisco, CA (109 cases); New York, NY (58); Jersey City, NJ (55); Newark, NY (50); Miami, FL (50); Fort Lauderdale, FL (50); and West Palm Beach, FL (40).

2 Regional trends
In figure 1, the increase in the percentage of all AIDS cases in the USA for regions outside of large MSAs is shown—an increase from 15.5% in 1981 to 35.3% in 1989. This trend affirms the assertion made by myself and others (Dutt et al, 1987), that the disease is spreading in a hierarchical pattern from higher central places (large cities) to lower ones (smaller cities). This trend also shows out that the disease is spreading outside of the homosexual populations concentrated in, for example, New York, San Francisco, and Los Angeles. There now appears to be a greatly increased chance of contracting the disease even if one does not belong to one of the groups originally regarded as at high risk and live in a large city. The percentage of AIDS cases in large MSAs has continued to decrease, whereas the percentage of cases outside large MSAs has steadily increased with the disbursement of the disease. A regional map based on the CDC data for urban areas with populations in excess of

1 000 000 has been provided (figure 2). We define regions as consisting of cities with populations over 1 000 000. Urban and other places with less than 1 000 000 people have been grouped into a not-large MSA (NLMSA) category, which has not been regionally differentiated.

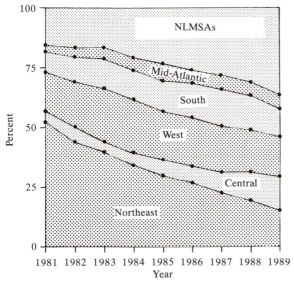

Figure 1. The percentage of new AIDS cases in the period 1981–89 for 5 regions (see figure 2); only cities with a population of over 1 000 000 have been included. The category 'NLMSAs' represents cities and places all over the USA which individually have populations of less than 1 000 000. Source: CDC, 1990.

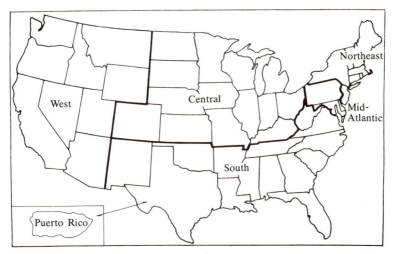

Figure 2. The 5 study regions, as based on data for urban places with populations in excess of 1 000 000. Source: CDC, 1990.

The increase in the percentage of AIDS cases outside large MSAs regardless of their racial mix shows the trend toward the disbursement of AIDS throughout the USA. Figure 3 points out that the proportion of AIDS victims among females and heterosexual males has increased recently, whereas the proportion of homosexual males with the disease has consistently declined during the 8-year (1981–89) span. Homosexuals, despite their reported high promiscuity (Dutt et al, 1987) have taken much greater precaution in their sexual intercourse and thus their rate of disease incidence is declining.

However, the virus is presumed to have spread rapidly in its beginnings because of the high density of sexually active homosexuals and of IV drug abusers in metropolitan areas (Altman, 1988; Joseph, 1988), and because the disease is still confined mainly to these two groups it is entering slowly into the rest of the population.

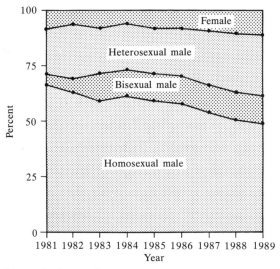

Figure 3. Percentile composition of new AIDS victims in the period 1981–89 by gender and by male sexuality. Source: CDC, 1990.

3 Patient groups

Known risk groups now include homosexuals, bisexuals, and IV drug abusers, and these account for 87% of the AIDS cases in the USA. This percentage has remained constant during recent years (*MMWR*, 1985). However, new risk groups seem to be developing as the disease spreads throughout the general population.

AIDS in the USA still largely affects homosexuals, bisexuals, and IV drug abusers (figure 3 and table 1). This statement applies to the nation as a whole, NLMSAs, or large MSAs of different regions of the country.

Whereas in 1981 71.9% of the victims were homosexual or bisexual men, the percentage had dropped to 62.1% in 1989 (table 1). Palca points out that such a dip "taken together with new surveillance data, has prompted epidemiologists to cut by approximately 15% the number of AIDS cases predicted over the next 3 years" (Palca, 1989, page 1560). Cases among IV drug abusers, however, have risen from 11.0% in 1981 to 23.5% in 1989. Though there has been a decrease in the proportion of homosexuals with AIDS, the increase in the proportion of IV drug abusers with AIDS since 1981 (Thomas, 1986) signals a shift toward an increased incidence among the rest of the population because infected IV drug abusers can spread the disease among formerly low-risk groups through heterosexual contact. In 1989, up to 26% of the AIDS transmission took place by heterosexual contacts. The percentile share of AIDS arising from blood transfusions, both for adults and for children, peaked in 1987 and thereafter sharply declined as a result of stricter detection procedures for the virus in the blood pool.

There is also an increasing percentage of female cases, arising from IV drug abuse and sexual contact with male IV drug abusers. More than three quarters of the cases in women patients involve IV drug abuse or sexual contact with men who are IV drug abusers (Thomas, 1986).

From figure 4, we can see that, proportionately, the Northeast has the highest percentage of its AIDS victims (dead or alive) among IV drug abusers, and the second-highest percentage is among homosexual and bisexual men. The places in the NLMSA category are spread throughout the country and have numbers of IV-drug-abusing AIDS victims second only to the Northeast. Thus, heterosexuals now risk contracting the disease throughout the country.

Curran et al (1988) pointed out that from 1982 to 1986 the proportion of AIDS cases caused by heterosexual transmission of AIDS doubled. The CDC statistics show that the proportion of heterosexual males and females with AIDS rose considerably from 1981 to 1989. The long-term

Table 1. Annual percentile composition of AIDS victims in the USA by patient group.

Group	1981	1982	1983	1984	1985	1986	1987	1988	1989
Male homosexual	65.2	60.3	61.2	64.1	64.1	63.1	60.4	56.5	56.3
IV drug abuser	11.0	16.9	17.7	16.7	17.5	17.9	19.9	22.8	23.5
Male bisexual	6.7	9.6	9.6	8.8	7.4	7.7	6.8	6.0	5.8
Haemophiliac	0.5	0.6	0.4	1.0	1.0	0.9	1.0	1.0	0.9
Heterosexual	0.5	1.1	0.9	1.4	1.9	2.4	3.1	4.0	4.3
Born with AIDS	6.1	4.9	3.6	2.2	1.6	1.4	1.2	1.1	1.3
Blood transfusion patient	0.5	1.0	1.5	1.7	2.4	2.7	2.8	2.5	1.5
Undetermined	4.3	2.9	2.5	2.3	2.1	2.4	3.2	4.7	5.6

consequences of this trend need to be taken seriously because there is a tendency for long periods to occur between infection with the virus and the onslaught of the opportunistic diseases (4–15 years), people infected with the virus may unknowingly be transmitting it for many years (Kung-Jong et al, 1988).

Sonoma in California may be experiencing the effects of this type of build up. With a large homosexual population and IV drug abusers, Sonoma has the second-highest number of cases per capita in the state. Since 1980, the number of cases has doubled. The formerly latent pool of the infection has built up over the years and is now being reflected in the number of cases occurring (Horowitz, 1987). The same is true of many other areas in the USA. The lengthy incubation period also puts blood-transfusion recipients at a high risk, because preventive screening measures were not instituted until 1985.

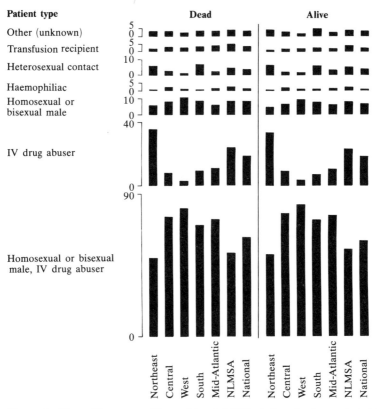

Figure 4. Percentile composition of total AIDS victims in the period 1981–89 by patient groups, based on the categories 'dead' and 'alive'. Figures to the left indicate the percentage of the total number of cases in the USA by region, NLMSAs (not-large Metropolitan Statistical Area), and for the nation. Source: CDC, 1990.

The number of AIDS patients in the IV drug abuse category who have
died could be higher than statistics show, because there is a controversy
about what the CDC says constitutes an AIDS-related death. Reclassification
would alter especially the number of black people reported to be
affected (Curran et al, 1988). Many deaths attributed to IV drug abuse
may be reclassified upon reexamination.

Some of the decline in the proportion of homosexual cases may be
due, in part, to changes in sexual practices. There has been much
information directed at the high-risk group of homosexuals, and this
trend may reflect an adjustment in their behaviour.

It seems that heterosexuals particularly females, may in the long run
become the main risk group of the disease. The virus is presumed to
have spread rapidly in the USA because of the high density of sexually
active homosexuals and IV drug abusers in metropolitan areas (Thomas,
1986). This is one of the reasons why the Northeast, centering around
the New York metropolitan area, has also the highest percentage share
of AIDS victims (table 2) in comparison with all other regions. It is in
this metropolitan area that there is a much higher proportion of black
people and Hispanics compared with the nation as a whole, and so these
two minority groups are in greater risk of contracting the disease,
particularly from sexual contact with IV drug abusers and their sexual
partners.

Table 2. Regional AIDS cases by race (%), 1981–88. Percentage figures are
calculated from the total of each racial group. Source: CDC, 1990.

Region	White	Black	Hispanic	Other
Large MSA				
Northeast	19.9	39.8	44.9	25.1
Central	7.4	6.6	3.1	3.8
West	28.8	8.6	16.4	41.3
South	14.2	11.2	12.3	3.7
Mid-Atlantic	5.4	10.7	1.8	1.5
NLMSA	24.2	23.0	21.3	24.5

Note: MSA, Metropolitan Statistical Area; NLMSA, not-large MSA.

4 Race
AIDS victims who have contracted the disease via a blood transfusion
are more prevalent among white (Caucasoid) people. Black (Negroid)
people and Hispanics have a much higher incidence of AIDS cases
arising from heterosexual contact compared with white people. There is
an unusually high incidence of AIDS transmitted by heterosexual contact
among black people in the Southern region, probably the result of the
connection with the disease in the Caribbean islands, where it is more
prevalent in the heterosexual population than in the homosexual population.

Except for in the NLMSAs, over 75% of white people with AIDS fall in
the category of homosexual or bisexual males in all 5 regions. In the
group of patients who are IV drug abusers, there is an unusually high
concentration of black people and Hispanics in the Northeast (figure 5).
The affliction of these minorities with the disease can be assessed from the
fact that in the year 1989, the annual rate of AIDS incidence for the nation
was 14.2 per 100 000 population, but among black people and Hispanics it
accounted for 34.7 and 26.3 per 100 000 population, respectively.

The distribution of AIDS victims by racial category in 1981 was
59.1% white, 25.4% black, and 14.7% Hispanic. The 1989 figures of
54.1% white people, 30.2% black people, and 14.5% Hispanic show a
significant shift in the increase of cases among black people. (Note: in
1989 white, black, and Hispanic people were estimated to constitute
80%, 11%, and 7% of the total US population, respectively.) This
increase can be attributed to the increase of black people with AIDS

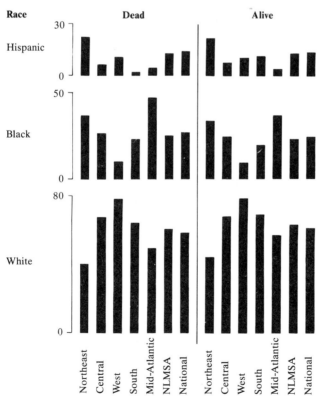

Figure 5. Percentile composition of AIDS victims in the period 1981–89 by
race, based on the categories 'dead' and 'alive'. Figures to the left indicate the
percentage of the total number of cases in the USA by region, NLMSAs (not-
large Metropolitan Statistical Areas), and for the nation. Source: CDC, 1990.

related to IV drug abuse (Curran et al, 1988). The decline of AIDS
cases among white people is related to the percentile decline in the
incidence among homosexuals; 80% of the homosexual or bisexual
contract cases in the USA in 1989 were white people.

Among white victims, both dead or alive, the Western region still has
the highest incidence at 28.8% (see table 2). The NLMSA accounts for the
next largest percentage among the white cases at 24.2%. Among black
people and Hispanics, the highest concentration of cases is in the
Northeast region, with, respectively, 36.8% and 39.8% of their national
prevalence of AIDS cases being located there. Until 1989, 29 742 male
AIDS patients were reported to belong to the heterosexual exposure
category; of which 36% consisted of black people and 21% of Hispanic
people (USDHE/CDC, 1990). A break up of the dead-or-alive status of
AIDS victims by region indicates that among black people, the number
of dead AIDS victims outnumbers those who are alive, and this is also
true of black victims in all the regions except the West (figure 5). Black
people have less access in general to costly medicines, and a large
number of them do not have private medical insurance with which to
take prompt advantage of health-care facilities.

5 Gender

Though female AIDS cases had been too low to report separately
before 1981, there is an alarming increase in numbers of women with
the disease. In 1981, only 33 victims were female (not including
children), but in 1988 the number rose to 1 806 (over the age of 14).
The increase of AIDS victims who are female appears to be related to
sexual contact with men who are IV drug abusers and to the incidence
of IV drug abuse by women (Altman, 1988).

This trend is significant because of the direct relationship of children
born with AIDS as a secondary result of maternal IV drug abuse or of
their mother's heterosexual activity with an IV drug abuser carrying the
virus. Because of the efficient nature of transmission from the maternal
blood supply to the foetus in utero or during birth when there is an
enhanced risk of exposure of the baby to maternal blood, the incidence
of perinatal transmission tends to be high (Lapointe et al, 1985). New
York City has a reported incidence of more than twice the national
average (reported at 7%) of infants born with AIDS: 16% (Joseph, 1988).

6 New groups of patients

The rapid increase in paediatric AIDS cases warrants the creation of a
separate category to track the increasing number of children born with
the disease. The parents of these children are mostly in the previously
described high-risk groups. There were only 19 AIDS cases in the 12-
years-and-under age-group in 1981, but in 1988 the total number of
victims rose to 1489, almost 2% of the total number of AIDS patients.

Of a total of 1995 paediatric (below the age of 13) AIDS cases reported through 1989, 52.6% are black, 24.6% Hispanic, and 21.8% white.

Among paediatric patients, the majority are black children, with one or both parents having AIDS or one or both parents being considered to be in a high-risk category. Among the AIDS victims who are less than a year old, 59.9% are black, 21.7% are Hispanic, and 17.5% are white. (Note: in 1989, white, black, and Hispanic children were estimated to constitute 75%, 14%, and 10% of the total US population under 5 years old, respectively.) In contrast, the lower incidence of white AIDS victims in the paediatric age-group is because these cases are still predominantly the outcome of homosexual contacts.

A total of 1 in 40 infants in the Bronx, New York, is born carrying the AIDS virus. It is predicted that by 1991, 10000 to 20000 children will be infected in the USA. It is also known that 90% of the children with AIDS also suffer some form of brain damage (Montgomery, 1989).

7 Death from AIDS
Table 3(a) shows the year of diagnosis and survival rate of AIDS patients. Roughly one third of the patients are dead within approximately 2 years of being diagnosed. Over 50% are dead within 3 years. More than

Table 3. The survival rate of AIDS patients (%), by (a) year (count taken in 1989), (b) gender, and (c) race. Source: CDC, 1990.

	Alive		Dead	
	percent	number	percent	number
(a) Year				
1981	11.0	41	89.0	333
1982	10.9	109	89.1	894
1983	9.4	274	90.6	2651
1984	14.0	882	86.0	5050
1985	16.7	1813	83.3	9049
1986	26.0	4528	74.0	12869
1987	45.1	11135	54.9	13543
1988	69.7	17765	30.3	17720
(b) Gender				
Male				
homosexual	44.6		55.4	
bisexual	44.1		55.9	
other	43.3		56.7	
Female	43.0		57.0	
(c) Race				
White	45.3		54.7	
Black	41.5		58.5	
Hispanic	43.8		56.2	
Others	49.0		51.0	

55.9% of the AIDS victims recorded in the period 1981–88 had died by 1988. This cumulative percentile share of dead will increase if AIDS remains uncurable. Table 3(b) shows the survival rate by gender. The male patient has a slightly higher survival rate (only by 1.6%) than the female patient. Table 3(c) shows the survival rate by race, with the white AIDS patients having a slightly better survival rate than black or Hispanic patients. 'Other' patients constitute less than 1% of the total AIDS victims and therefore are not discussed here. This finding might reflect the better medical care that can be afforded by many of the white patients and also may be influenced by health problems associated with IV drug abuse in the black and Hispanic populations (Curran et al, 1988). In 1986, AIDS was the leading cause of death of haemophiliacs and IV drug abusers in the USA (Curran et al, 1988). Most children that are born with AIDS die within 3 years. Especially hard hit is New York, where three-quarters of the children with AIDS have died (Joseph, 1988).

8 AIDS patients by country of birth

AIDS in the USA originated from a Haitian connection, possibly reinforced from Central Africa and the Caribbean islands, including the West Indies. The disease was carried by homosexuals from Haiti where there was a large homosexual population during the late 1970s and early 1980s.

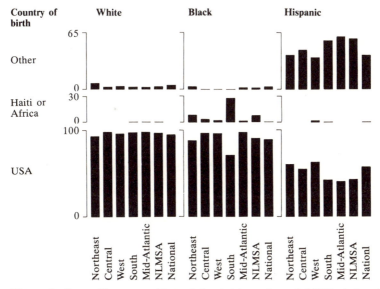

Figure 6. Percentile composition of the total number of AIDS victims by country of birth within the categories black, white, and for the racial group of Hispanics for the period 1981–89. Figures to the left indicate the percentage of the total number of cases by region, NLMSA (not-large Metropolitan Statistical Area), and for the nation. Source: CDC, 1990.

However, the Central African and Caribbean carriers were generally heterosexuals. The US victims born in Haiti or Central Africa constituted up to 6.4% of the total AIDS victims in 1981 (figure 6). As time passed, the percentile share of US-born victims increased, from 83.7% in 1981 to 92.7% in 1989. Similarly, the percentile share of victims born in other countries, excluding Haiti, dropped from 9.9% to 1981 to 5.9% in 1989.

A high proportion of white AIDS victims in the USA are US born (96.4%), the Hispanic victims are nearly all foreign born (figure 6). Among the black victims, the Southern region has a high proportion (28%) who were born in Haiti and Central Africa. One of the reasons that black and Hispanic people have a much higher proportion of victims in the heterosexual contact group of AIDS patients is that they have a disease linkage with the Caribbean islands and Central Africa, where the disease is predominantly transmitted by heterosexual contact. Among all the heterosexual patients in the USA, 49.9% are black and 23.1% Hispanic. White people constitute 57.1% of the total AIDS victims, and form 29% of the heterosexual patients.

9 Changing risk groups
In the early 1980s, homosexuals predominated as the main AIDS risk group in the USA (figure 7) and the Haitian connection was playing the main role in its diffusion. The disease had entered the pool of IV drug abusers through homosexual or bisexual AIDS victims by the mid-1980s. Through the IV drug abusers, bisexual, and heterosexual out-of-country AIDS victims, the disease entered into the heterosexual population at an increasing rate. By 1990, the disease had diffused into a wider group of the population, though the domination of homosexual or bisexual male victims continued. The IV drug abusers became the group with the fastest rate of increase. Other new groups on the increase included the paediatric and female heterosexual groups. Thus heterosexuals might

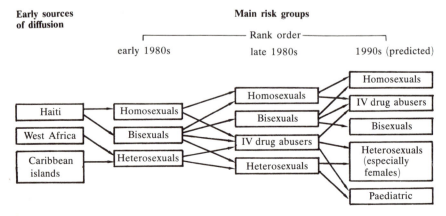

Figure 7. Sources and changes in the AIDS risk groups in the USA.

ultimately play a larger role in the spread of the disease if the pace of disease growth remains unchecked. Recent statistics point to a drop in the rate of increase of AIDS in the USA, and some attribute the dip to the effect of therapy and to a decrease in the rate of HIV transmission from earlier years (Palca, 1989).

10 Conclusions and speculations
The patterns and trends that reflect the increase of AIDS in the population require attention by health-care officials. AIDS continues to be a fatal disease with no known cure. What is especially disturbing is that the virus appears to be developing resistance to Azidothymidine (AZT), the only known drug that offers any relief from the AIDS symptoms (Palca, 1990).

Everyone must become educated to the risks which may expose them to AIDS and the preventive behaviour that may be taken, especially in consideration of the new trends and patient types and the impact these trends may have on society. Government and private-sector institutions may not be able to handle the epidemic if it spreads too rapidly.

As research proceeds to find effective treatment, a cure, and vaccine, more evidence suggests that it may be even harder than previously realised. This problem arises because of the nature of the AIDS virus itself. Its genetic variability helps it to escape the human immune system and greatly complicates any development of vaccines (*Science*, 1988). Nevertheless, it was reported in December 1989 that researchers at Tulane University (New Orleans, Louisiana) had discovered a vaccine that has been successful in tests on monkeys. If proven successful on humans, a test which is imminent, there will be a revolutionary change in controlling the disease, not only in the USA but all over the world.

Acknowledgements. M Gargaret Geib (cartographer) and Xchun Xie (visiting scholar), both of the University of Akron, are thanked for preparing the diagrams and assisting in the computer analysis, respectively.

References
Altman R, 1988, "The epidemiology of AIDS in New Jersey" *New York State Journal of Medicine* **88** 236–238
Brooke J, 1989, "Rapid spread of AIDS alarms the Ivory Coast" *The New York Times, International* 12 March, page 12
CDC, 1990, AIDS Case Reports, Publication Information Data Tape, January, Centers for Disease Control; available at Center for Infectious Diseases, Division of HIV/AIDS, Centers for Disease Control, Atlanta, GA 30333
Curran J W, Jaffe H W, Hardy A M, Morgan W M, Selik R M, Dondero T J, 1988, "Epidemiology of HIV infection and AIDS in the United States" *Science* **239** 610–616
Dutt A K, Monroe C, Dutta H M, Prince B, 1987, "Geographical patterns of AIDS in the United States" *Geographical Review* **77** 456–471
Horowitz N, 1987, "AIDS in S.F. exurbia, not N.Y.C. exurbia" *Medical Tribune* 1 April

Joseph S C, 1988, "Current issues concerning AIDS in New York City" *New York State Journal of Medicine* **88** 253–258

Jovaisas E, Koch M A, Schäfer A, Stauber M, Löwenthal D, 1985, "LAV/HTLV-III in 20-week fetus" *Lancet* **ii**

Koop C E, 1989, "Responding to the patient who has AIDS" *Journal of the American Medical Colleges* **64** 113

Kung-Jong L, Darrow W W, Rutherford G W, 1988, "A model-based estimate of the mean incubation period for AIDS in homosexual men" *Science* **240** 1333–1335

Lapointe N, Michaud J, Pekovic D, Chausseau J P, Dupuy J, 1985, "Transplacemental transmission of HTLV-III virus" *New England Journal of Medicine* **312** 1325

MMWR 1985, "Heterosexual transmission of human T-cell lymphotropic virus type III/lymphadeopathy-associated virus" *Morbidity and Mortality Weekly Report* **34** Number 3Y 561–563

MMWR 1986, "Update: acquired immunodeficiency syndrome—United States" *Morbidity and Mortality Weekly Report* **35**(2) 17 January, pages 17–21

Montgomery G, 1989, "The Infant Brain" *Discover* **10**(8) 30–32 (available from Family Media Inc., 3 Park Avenue, New York, NY10016, USA)

Palca J, 1989, "Is the AIDS epidemic slowing?" *Science* **246** (22 December) 1560

Palca J, 1990, "Trials and tribulations of AIDS drug testing" *Science* **247** (23 March) 1406

Science 1988, "The AIDS virus can take on many guises" **241** (26 August) 1039–1040

Selik R M, Haverkos H W, Curran J W, 1984, "Acquired immune deficiency syndrome (AIDS) trends in the United States, 1978–1982" *American Journal of Medicine* **76** 493–500

Shannon G W, Pyle G F, 1989, "The origin and diffusion of AIDS: a view from medical geography" *Annals of the Association of American Geographers* **79** 1–24

Thomas P, 1986, "The AIDS epidemic in New York City, 1981–84" *American Journal of Epidemiology* **123** 1013–1025

USDHE/CDC, 1990 *HIV/AIDS Surveillance Report* January, US Department of Health and Education/Centers for Disease Control, Atlanta, GA 30333, pages 1–22

Part 4

Mental Health and the Environment

Pathways to Mental Care: The Role of the General Practitioner in Salford

S SCOBIE
University of Manchester

1 Introduction

The deinstitutionalisation of psychiatric patients to forms of community care has formed an important element of health care policy in many Western countries since the early 1960s. Subsequently, much research has been devoted to problems stemming from both the readjustment of patients to life in the community, and the reactions of residents to new treatment facilities in the community (Smith and Giggs, 1988). A natural outcome of such a policy would be to expect a substantial reduction in the numbers of patients in institutional (inpatient) care. However, recent studies (Nutter and Thomas, 1990; Wooff et al, 1983) based on the Salford Psychiatric Case Register reveal only a small decline in the numbers of inpatients, but indicate large increases (more than 50% between 1978 and 1985) in prevalence for patients using all psychiatric services. This figure excludes patients treated by their general practitioner (GP).

It is possible that such growth might reflect a genuine increase in the prevalence of mental disorder in Salford. Conversely, this outcome might simply be a function of the improved detection of illness, associated with the provision of new services such as the community psychiatric nurse (CPN). In this paper, I examine some facets of this problem, and am concerned with the relationships between facility location and usage. In particular, I analyse the role of the GP as a filter between illness in the community and treatment at specialised psychiatric agencies. My central concern is to explain variations in the referral of psychiatric disorders among Salford's GPs in relation to the organisation, size, and social composition of their practices.

In the following discussion, the factors influencing the pathway to psychiatric care are reviewed. In particular, a patient's GP is shown to play a central role in the referral process, and the current contribution of primary care services to the care of the mentally ill is discussed. Following this, the factors affecting referral which have been included in this analysis are presented, and their influence, both individually and together, is analysed. Last, the implications for the provision of services to the mentally ill are evaluated, particularly in the light of recent developments in health policy.

2 Mental illness in general practice

Studies of mental illness in the community have shown that only a minority of people with psychological disorders reach specialist care (Shepherd et al, 1966). As awareness of the extent of untreated mental illness has grown, the role of the referral system in selecting some of the many mentally ill people for treatment has become apparent (Goldberg and Huxley, 1980). Patients reaching specialist care have in many cases been referred to a psychiatrist by their GP, although some patients may reach care through social services, community nursing, or hospital emergency services.

Goldberg and Huxley have developed a model for understanding the referral process through the patient's GP. This is seen as a series of filters through which the patient must pass in order to reach successive levels of care (figure 1). At each stage the patient's chances of passing the filter depend to some extent on the character and severity of the illness, but also on the patient's social and demographic attributes, on the GP's ability to detect the illness and confidence to treat it, and on the services available to patient and GP.

The first filter in the model is the decision to consult. Studies of help-seeking for physical illness suggest that in order for need for a service to become demand, the individual must first recognise her or his need, must be aware that help is available to meet this need, and must then be able to meet the service (Mechanic, 1982). Despite these intervening factors, surveys of psychiatric morbidity in the community and among people visiting their GP suggest that the majority of those with mental illness, between 80% and 90%, do consult their GP (Brown and Harris, 1978; Hagnell, 1966; Weissman and Myers, 1978). However, many people consult with physical complaints, and have not identified themselves as being in need of psychiatric care (Fitzpatrick et al, 1984; Good, 1977).

The second filter in the model is the ability of GPs to detect the illness. Approximately a half of cases of psychiatric disorder are missed by GPs (Freeling et al, 1985; Goldberg and Blackwell, 1970). The characteristics and interviewing style of the GP affect the GP's accuracy and bias in detecting mental illness (Davenport et al, 1987; Goldberg and Huxley, 1980). Goldberg et al (1980) identified a number of factors in a multivariate analysis of GP characteristics which were associated, to differing degrees, with their psychiatric assessments. First, GPs with a 'psychiatric emphasis', who ask many psychiatric questions and questions about the patient's home life, identify psychiatric disorders in more patients, but their assessments were not particularly accurate. Second, GPs with good interviewing techniques, and those with accurate concepts of psychiatric illness who ask directive questions, tended to make accurate assessments. Other significant factors were the academic ability and self-confidence of the doctor. Characteristics of the patient have also been found to be important: psychiatric disorders are less likely to be detected in patients who present with a physical complaint, and the patient's sociodemographic characteristics are significant.

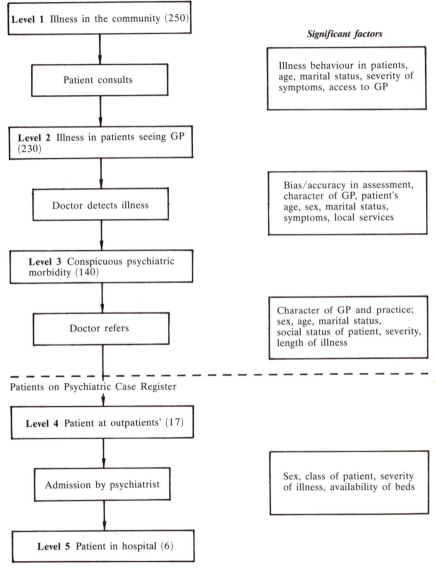

Figure 1. The pathway to psychiatric care. (Adapted from Goldberg and Huxley, 1980.) Note: numbers in brackets represent the number of people per 1000 population at risk.

The third filter to the use of psychiatric services is the decision of the GP to refer the patient to a specialist. Goldberg and Huxley found that at this stage the GP's confidence and ability to treat the case were important, as were the characteristics of the patient and the severity of the disorder (Goldberg and Huxley, 1980). Studies have found that patients with fewer social contacts are referred more often (Munk-Jorgensen, 1986), and that the social class of the patient is also important (Hurry et al, 1980). The majority of patients seen by GPs are suffering from nonpsychotic disorders, and most cases are not severe (Jenkins and Shepherd, 1983). Cases of above-average severity are more likely to be referred, and psychotic patients are almost certain to reach specialist care eventually. However, a significant minority of depressed patients in primary care have severe disorders, and there is concern that the needs of these patients are poorly served in general practice (Blacker and Clare, 1987).

The management of psychiatric disorder in primary care shows wide variation between practitioners, with regard to referral to specialists and to prescribing habits. However, the reasons for these differences are not clear. A study of urban general practices in Manchester found no significant association between the characteristics of GPs and their management of psychosocial illness (Whitehouse, 1987). Wide variation in referral rates have been found for other specialties (Dowie, 1983), but again, the characteristics of GPs have largely failed to explain differences in referral rates (Wilkin and Smith, 1987).

The influence of service availability on referral is unclear. Goldberg and Huxley suggest that the availability of services is only a weak influence on referral, although GPs were influenced by whether or not the specialist services would be acceptable to the patient, in terms of access but also with respect to the patient's perception of these services. GPs in this and other studies (Tryer, 1985) were aware of the stigma attached to psychiatric care, which would make referral to a specialist an unacceptable option for some patients. In addition, a recent review of referral practices indicates that a community-oriented service leads to higher rates of referrals (Wilkinson, 1989). The potential impact of specialist services on referral rates is acquiring increasing importance as more services are provided in primary care settings. In response to growing awareness of the vital role of GPs in the care of the chronically ill (HCSSSC, 1985), attempts have been made to develop ways of improving treatment in primary care settings. The roles of consultant psychiatrists (Tryer, 1985; Williams and Balestrieri, 1989), CPNs (Ginnsberg et al, 1984), therapists (Wilson and Wilson, 1985), and social workers (Corney, 1984) in primary care have all been evaluated at one time or another. Although all kinds of intervention prove beneficial to some patients, important problems exist for their routine use with respect to selecting which patients will benefit and to assess the reduction, if any, in demand on GPs.

A central problem is whether the provision of services in primary care settings reduces demand for hospital-based services, as intended. However, primary care provision can also increase demand in two ways: first, by adding an extra level of service provision for patients who will go on to use hospital services anyway; and second, by increasing the referral of patients who would not have reached specialist care. Williams and Balestrieri (1989) identified a negative correlation between clinics in general practice and admissions, suggesting that clinics are an alternative to hospital care. However, other studies have found that psychiatric clinics in general practice increase the referral of patients to specialists, by an estimated 19% (Tryer, 1985), because the service is easier to use and there is an absence of stigma. An increase in overall referrals, however, can occur along with a fall in admissions to hospital (Tryer et al, 1989).

In a comparison of referral in 6 urban health districts (Whitehouse, 1987) it was found that referral to nursing staff was higher in one district with a well-developed CPN service, but this did not reduce referrals to consultants. A similar scenario is suggested by the studies of the CPN service in Salford (Wooff and Goldberg, 1988; Wooff et al, 1986; 1988), where use of this service is not associated with a reduction in the uptake of hospital services. Wooff and her colleagues found that as the CPN service in Salford expanded, the proportion of schizophrenics, for whom the service was initially planned, decreased and CPNs were increasingly treating depressed patients. Patients seeing only CPNs accounted for a substantial portion of the increase in prevalence rates during the period of study, and it was concluded that CPNs were treating primary care patients, rather than offering extramural services to chronic psychotic patients (Wooff et al, 1986).

3 Research design

In the analysis which follows, the factors which influence the pathway to specialist psychiatric services in Salford are explored. A range of potentially important factors have been identified during the preceding discussion: the characteristics of general practice, the social characteristics of patients, and the provision of specialist services. These variables have been used in this analysis, with use of the measures discussed below. Unfortunately, no information about 'true' levels of psychiatric disorder among patients in general practice is available, and the variation in GP referral behaviour cannot be distinguished from variation in the underlying need of patients or from the differences in detection rates between GPs. However, reference will be made to the social characteristics of the practice, to reduce this confounding influence.

Data were drawn from the Salford Psychiatric Case Register, in which all contacts of Salford residents with the psychiatric services are recorded.

Incidence cases for the 3-year period 1980–82 have been analysed: these are patients with no known history of using psychiatric services who first contacted the psychiatric services in 1980–82. The analysis covers incidence cases from the whole of Salford, although GPs and their patients have been excluded if the GP was not on the list of the Salford Family Practitioner Committee for a complete year during the period under study. This list also excludes GPs with practices outside of Salford, even if they were treating Salford patients. Approximately 10% of inceptors in 1980–82 did not have a GP eligible for inclusion in this investigation, including some patients whose GP was not known from the Psychiatric Case Register or could not be traced through the records of the Family Practitioner Committee. In all, 2782 of the 3129 cases have been included. Patients who were not included do not differ in their social or demographic characteristics from other cases.

The Psychiatric Case Register records each patient's GP, and incidence rates have been calculated for GP premises: the analysis has been conducted on the basis of premises rather than individual GPs, because the list size of GPs in group practice does not always reflect their actual workload[1] (Wilkin and Metcalfe, 1984). The average list size of each GP for complete years of practice has been used to calculate the number of patients at each GP premises. Incidence cases have likewise been amalgamated to GP premises.

These incidence rates have been compared with the characteristics of general practice and the availability of services to the GP. The provision of specialist services to the premises is recorded: whether or not the premises had a consultant outpatient clinic or CPN staff attached to it, and the number of CPNs who were working from the premises. All 7 health centres had CPNs working from them at some time during 1980–82. In addition, between 2 and 3 CPNs worked in the Little Hulton/Walkden area, working from offices at Peel Hall Hospital and Park Clinic in Walkden. A total of 6 health centres had consultant outpatient clinics and these are indicated in table 1. The extent of outpatient provision varied between health centres and over time, and it is recognised that the presence of a clinic will not be a particularly sensitive measure of the availability of services.

Other characteristics of the GP's practice have also been included: whether the practice is in a health centre, the number of GPs working at the premises, and the average list size of GPs at the premises. There are 126 GPs included in the study, working from 51 premises, and these premises are shown in figure 2, along with the hospitals, health

---

[1] A number of difficulties were encountered with the list of GPs practising in Salford, and it has not been possible to identify which GPs were in group practice and with whom. The allocation of GPs to premises has been undertaken on the basis of their addresses, and does not necessarily imply a partnership.

Table 1. The provision of specialist services in primary care settings.

	CPN staffing levels[a]			Outpatient clinic?
	1980	1981	1982	
Peel Hall/Park clinic	2.00	2.75	2.25	no
Ordsall HC	2.00	2.50	2.00	yes
Lance Burn HC	2.00	2.00	1.75	yes
Swinton and Pendlebury HC	2.00	2.00	2.00	yes
Lower Broughton HC	2.00	2.00	1.00	yes
Higher Broughton HC	0.00	0.00	1.00	no
Irlam	1.00	1.00	1.50	yes
Eccles	1.00	1.00	1.00	yes
Langworthy clinic	1.00	1.00	1.00	no

[a] CPNs taking training courses and the staffing input from the CPN organiser have been excluded from these figures.
Note: CPN community psychiatric nurse, HC health centre.

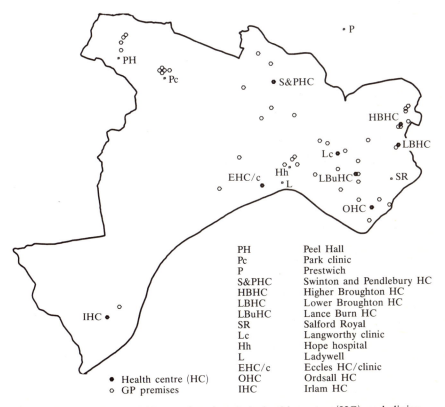

PH — Peel Hall
Pc — Park clinic
P — Prestwich
S&PHC — Swinton and Pendlebury HC
HBHC — Higher Broughton HC
LBHC — Lower Broughton HC
LBuHC — Lance Burn HC
SR — Salford Royal
Lc — Langworthy clinic
Hh — Hope hospital
L — Ladywell
EHC/c — Eccles HC/clinic
OHC — Ordsall HC
IHC — Irlam HC

● Health centre (HC)
○ GP premises

Figure 2. The location of GP premises, hospitals, health centres (HC), and clinics with community psychiatric nurses in the Salford medical district.

centres, and CPN offices in Salford. The list size and number of GPs
working at each practice is similar to that found in other studies of
urban general practice, although there is a slight preponderance of larger
practices, but a smaller average list size (Wilkin et al, 1987). GP
premises appear to be evenly distributed over Salford, the exceptions
being Kersal and Blackfriars, neither of which has a GP practice.

The social characteristics of the GPs' practices are represented by the
'super profile group' social area code (Brown and Batey, 1987). The 'super

Table 2. Amalgamated super profile groups (ASPGs).

Description of ASPG

ASPG 1: *White-collar group*
Mature professional and managerial families, semirural and suburban detached
    property.
Younger professional and managerial families, suburban detached and larger
    semidetached property.
Younger professional and white-collar families, suburban semidetached property.
Mixed, largely white-collar families in average-sized semidetached property.
High concentration of 1-person and 2-person pensioner households in owner-
    occupied property in white-collar groups.
1-person and 2-person professional and white-collar households, high proportion
    of students.

ASPG 2: *Mixed-social and housing group*
Skilled and semiskilled families, average unemployment, generally improved
    terraced housing.
Large young families containing semiskilled and unskilled workers in cramped
    owner-occupied and terraced property.
White-collar families together with some single workers. Widespread conversion
    of property to rented bedsits.
Young families, including a mixture of white-collar and blue-collar workers living
    in a mixture of owner-occupied and rented property.
Military bases, younger families, very high residential turnover.
All other areas—unclassified.

ASPG 3: *Council-housing and deprived group*
Unskilled families, high unemployment, flats in converted property.
Mixture of skilled and unskilled blue-collar workers, above-average unemployment,
    council housing, low residential turnover.
Older skilled and unskilled blue-collar workers, council housing, low residential
    turnover.
1-person and 2-person older households, council flats, low residential turnover.
Young skilled and semiskilled large families, council property, low residential
    turnover.
Unskilled families, high unemployment, ethnic groups, council flats.
Unskilled families, often with only 1 parent, high unemployment and average
    residential turnover.
Larger unskilled families, extremely high unemployment, very cramped council
    flats.

profile groups' have been amalgamated into 3 groups comprising white-collar areas, mixed areas, and areas with predominantly council housing. The composition of the 3 groups is shown in table 2. It is realised that the characteristics of the population in the immediate environs of the practice will not necessarily be shared by people on the GP's list. However, attempts to delimit the catchment area of GPs are fraught with difficulties because these areas are poorly defined (Wilkin et al, 1987).

A further 2 aspects of general practice were considered for inclusion: the spatial accessibility of the patient to the GP, and the spatial accessibility of the GP to hospital services and health centres. The former is known to affect attendance at primary care (Parkin, 1979; Phillips, 1981). However, its effect will be less important for patients with psychosocial problems, because such a high proportion of this group visit their GP, and distance to the GP premises has not been included in this analysis. The effect of proximity of the GP to hospitals and health centres has received little attention elsewhere, and distance measures to services have therefore been included. However, it is realised that their impact may be dwarfed by the role that organisational factors and personal contacts play in the referral process between GPs and specialists.

The incidence cases have been subdivided by diagnosis and type of care at inception, and the categories used are shown in table 3. Not all patients will have been referred to the psychiatric services by their GP, although this will be true for the majority. Patients whose first contact is a hospital emergency or a social worker are least likely to have been referred by their GP. Where reference to studies of referral are made in the discussion of the results, it must be borne in mind that the incidence rates discussed here are not directly comparable with GP referrals.

Table 3. Diagnostic and care groups.

Name	Description
SCHIZ	Schizophrenia
DEPR	Depression
DEM	Dementia
PERSD	Personality disorders
ANX	Anxiety disorders
AA	Alcoholism and addictions
TSD	Transient situational disturbance[a]
IP	Inpatient
OP	Outpatient
SW	Social work
CPN	Community psychiatric nurse
DOM	Domiciliary visit
EMER	Hospital emergency

[a] This diagnosis is given to patients with no previous history of mental illness who are suffering from stress-related psychological problems.

4 Patterns of incidence in Salford

4.1 Spatial variation and social factors

Incidence rates have been mapped with use of class intervals based on
nested means. Rates vary widely between GP premises, and as the class
intervals indicate, the distribution of rates is heavily skewed, with a
small number of GPs with very high rates. The wide variation in rates
is comparable with that found in the studies of referral which were
discussed earlier (see section 2).

A clear spatial pattern does not emerge from the mapping of most
diagnosis and care groups (figure 3), although a concentration of high-
incidence practices in the inner city can be discerned for anxiety
disorders, personality disorders, addictions, and transient situational
disturbance (not illustrated). GPs in Little Hulton also have high
incidence rates, particularly for depression and anxiety disorders.
Dementias are concentrated in the central area of Salford County
Borough. The spatial variation in rates for GP premises is consistent
with the association between high incidence and social deprivation,
which was explored in previous work in Salford (Scobie, 1989). However,

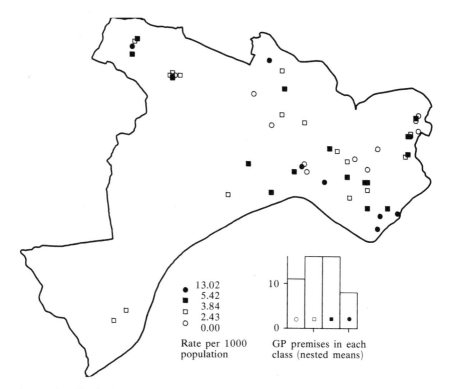

Figure 3. The incidence of psychiatric disorders (rate for GP practices 1980–82)
in Salford medical district.

the pattern is more diffuse, reflecting the wide variation between GPs, and, possibly, the low level of aggregation of cases. A comparison of rates for premises in different amalgamated super profile groups (figure 4) indicates higher rates at premises in socially deprived areas for some diagnoses and care groups, but the trend is far from uniform.

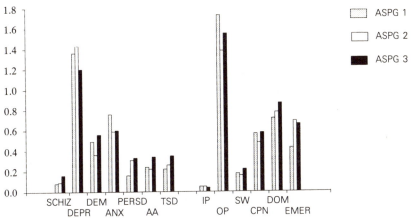

Figure 4. Mean rate of referral per 1000 GP patients by social area of premises. (See table 3 for description of care groups.) For definition of amalgamated super profile groups (ASPGs) see table 2.

4.2 Provision of specialist services

The pattern of incidence varies with the characteristics of the premises, and high incidence is associated with GPs in health centres, premises with CPNs attached, and those where an outpatient clinic is held (table 4). These three aspects of primary care provision are themselves closely related: all the health centres have CPNs attached, and all the premises with outpatient clinics are health centres. Their effects are not uniform over diagnostic and care groups, as is indicated in figure 5, and the

Table 4. Mean incidence rates per 1000 GP patients.

Premises	All cases		CPN inceptors excluded?	
	no	yes	no	yes
CPNs attached	3.73 ($n = 43$)	4.34 ($n = 8$)	3.28	3.30
Health centres	3.74 ($n = 44$)	4.44 ($n = 7$)	3.28	3.30
Outpatient clinic	3.72 ($n = 45$)	4.68 ($n = 6$)	3.25	3.51

Note: CPN community psychiatric nurse.

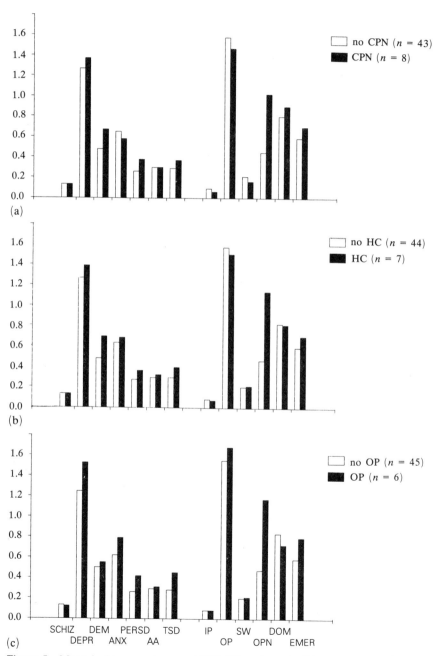

Figure 5. Mean incidence rates per 1000 GP patients in (a) premises with and without community psychiatric nurses (CPNs), (b) premises in health centres (HCs), and (c) premises with and without an outpatient clinic (OP).

differences between mean rates are small or negligible for most groups, the exception being the rate for CPN inceptors. The difference in rates for outpatient inceptors is less clear-cut: rates are lower for premises with CPNs and those in health centres, but higher when only premises with outpatient clinics are considered.

The higher rate of CPN inceptors in certain premises suggests that the presence of this service in primary care might increase incidence. When inceptions to CPNs are excluded the rates for premises in each group are similar (table 4), indicating that incidences in non-CPN services are not reduced by the availability of CPN staff at GP premises. The role of outpatient clinics is less clear, although the higher inception rates of outpatients in premises with outpatient clinics, compared with the lower rates for CPN clinics, is a weak indication that clinics influence the pattern of inceptions. The correlations between rates for each care group are weak in most cases (table 5). This suggests that the variation does not arise from high-referring and low-referring GPs, but possibly from selective referral to certain services. However, the spatial accessibility to services does not appear to be important, and rates are unrelated to distance of the premises to hospitals (Scobie, 1989).

The number of GPs at the premises was compared with incidence rates, but it appears that there is no consistent association between large practices and high rates, and although the very large practices have higher rates, these are health centres, and have specialist services at the premises. A more detailed study of GP behaviour would be needed to clarify this issue. However, higher incidence at group practices would be inconsistent with previous studies of referral which have found that solo GPs refer more patients (Wilkinson, 1989).

Table 5. Correlation between incidence rates for type of care groups[a].

	IP	OP	SW	CPN	DOM	EMER
IP	1.00	−0.07	0.12	−0.16	0.08	0.32
OP	−0.07	1.00	0.36	0.31	0.53	0.09
SW	0.12	0.36	1.00	0.25	0.60	0.19
CPN	−0.16	0.31	0.25	1.00	0.17	0.07
DOM	0.08	0.53	0.60	0.17	1.00	0.09
EMER	0.32	0.09	0.19	0.07	0.09	1.00

[a] For definition of care groups, see table 3.

5 Multivariate analysis of influences on incidence rates

The factors identified in the previous section—the social characteristics of the area, availability of a CPN service, and list size—may not be acting independently. The health centres and premises with CPNs attached are concentrated in socially disadvantaged areas of Salford (6 of the 7 health centres are in the third amalgamated super profile group) and this may contribute to the differences in rates. A further possible confounding influence is the social or academic characteristics of GPs who opt to work in group practice rather than singly, and in a health centre rather than in their own premises. It is possible that the observed differences are a result of the distribution and characteristics of GPs. The overlap between premises in health centres and those with CPNs or clinics is difficult to disentangle, because of the small number of premises involved.

To assess the relative importance of the main factors that were identified, a series of multiple regression models were estimated by using the independent variables listed in table 6 to predict the incidence of all illnesses (TOT) and each of the diagnostic categories listed in table 3. The independent variables denoting the presence of a CPN at a practice and its social area status were entered as dummy variables. The multiple regression equations (table 7) were constructed by using the stepwise procedure (Shaw and Wheeler, 1985) where independent variables are included in the equation only if their entry reduces the standard error of the forecast. This procedure did not always produce a significant level of explanation of the variation in the incidence rate $[p(F) \leqslant 0.05)]$, although the insignificant models for schizophrenia, dementia, and transient situational disturbance have been listed for reference. In table 7 the values of the partial regression coefficients of the independent variables included in each model are recorded, together with the exact significance of their t-ratios. The β weights enable comparison of the partial regression coefficients and indicate the change in the incidence rate generated by a standardised increment in each independent variable when all the others are controlled.

List size emerges from the analysis as the dominant influence on incidence rates, and is the only independent variable to exhibit significant partial regression coefficients for more than one diagnosis $[p(F) \leqslant 0.05]$. The incidence of all cases (TOT) fell with the average length of list, and there are significant variations amongst the diagnostic groups. The β weights for anxiety disorders (-0.49) and alcoholism/addictions (-0.43) are much lower than the weight for all cases (-0.36), indicating the

Table 6. Independent variables used in the regression analyses.

Name	Description
AVLIST	average list size of GPs in premises
CPN0	premises without CPN
CPN1	premises with CPN
ASPG1	premises in ASPG area 1
ASPG2	premises in ASPG area 2
ASPG3	premises in ASPG area 3

Note: GP general practitioner, CPN community psychiatric nurse, ASPG amalgamated super profile group.

strong impact of list size on the referral of these groups. The weight for depression (− 0.39) reveals a similar, although less-pronounced tendency. All these relationships probably reflect the association that has been established between list size and the average length of consultation time (Wilkin and Metcalfe, 1984). Longer consultation times have been linked to higher numbers of psychiatric assessments by GPs (Marks et al, 1979; Whitehouse, 1987), and to greater attention being paid to psychosocial problems.

Table 7. Stepwise multiple regressions: partial regression coefficients (b), β weights (given in parentheses), and goodness-of-fit statistics.

Ind. variable	TOT[a]		DEPR[a]		SCHIZ[a]		DEM[a]	
	b	S	b	S	b	S	b	S
AVLIST	−0.00011 (−0.36)	0.011	−0.00006 (−0.39)	0.008	−0.00001 (−0.19)	0.187	−	−
CPN0	−	−	−	−	−	−	−	−
CPN1	−	−	−	−	−	−	0.16975 (0.20)	0.159
ASPG1	−	−	−	−	−	−	−	−
ASPG2	−	−	−	−	−	−	−	−
ASPG3	−	−	−0.44297 (−0.19)	0.181	−	−	−	−
R^2	0.130		0.150		0.037		0.042	
F	7.001	0.011	4.051	0.024	1.794	0.187	2.053	0.159
df_r	1		2		1		1	
df_e	47		46		47		47	

	ANX[a]		PERSD[a]		AA[a]		TSD[a]	
	b	S	b	S	b	S	b	S
AVLIST	−0.00005 (−0.49)	0.001	−	−	−0.00002 (−0.43)	0.002	−0.00001 (−0.19)	0.194
CPN0	−	−	−	−	−	−	−	−
CPN1	0.16975 (0.20)	0.159	−	−	−	−	−	−
ASPG1	−	−	−0.17782 (0.32)	0.024	−	−	−	−
ASPG2	−	−	−	−	−	−	−	−
ASPG3	−0.29308 (−0.19)	0.157	−	−	−	−	−0.14220 (0.26)	0.078
R^2	0.224		0.104		0.185		0.080	
F	6.643	0.003	5.546	0.024	10.702	0.002	2.012	0.145
df_r	2		1		1		2	
df_e	46		47		47		46	

− Coefficients not listed because the standard error of the forecast increases if the variable is included.
[a] Dependent variable.
Note: S exact significance; TOT total; for definitions of the dependent and independent variables, see tables 3 and 6.

The insignificant relationships between list size and the incidence of both schizophrenia and dementia suggests the symptoms of these severe disorders are more easily recognised by the GP. In addition, almost all cases of schizophrenia will eventually come into contact with the psychiatric services, and therefore the filters to service use which operate in general practice are unlikely to exert a strong influence on recorded incidence of schizophrenia. It is worth noting that transient situational disturbance is the only disorder to reveal a positive, although insignificant, relationship with list size $[p(t_b) = 0.194]$. This result reflects the pathway to care taken by these patients, the majority of whom reach the psychiatric services after a hospital emergency, so bypassing primary care services.

The presence of a CPN is insignificant in all the regression models, although a weak positive relationship is recorded for the incidence of dementia $[p(t_b) = 0.159]$. This association is consistent with existing research on psychogeriatric services in Salford (Scobie, 1989), which has found that the provision of new services has led to large increases in demand from elderly patients.

Similarly, social area does not make a major contribution to the regression models. A weak negative association is observed between low status areas and depression $[p(t_b) = 0.181]$, anxiety disorders $[p(t_b) = 0.157]$, and transient situation disturbance $[p(t_b) = 0.078]$. In contrast, personality disorders are negatively related to high status areas $[p(t_b) = 0.024]$.

6 Conclusion

A number of influences on incidence have been considered, and the dominant relationships are the negative associations between list size and the incidence rates for many disorders. The presence of a CPN service at a premise increased the incidence of dementia diagnoses only, although this effect was generally weak. However, there was a much higher rate of incidence with the CPN service at premises where a CPN was present. This increase was not offset by lower rates for other services, a finding which is consistent with previous studies of the CPN service in Salford, which have linked the expansion of the service to higher demand for care (Wooff et al, 1986).

However, there was wide variation in incidence between GPs, and the factors discussed above explain only a small part of this variation. The differences in incidence rates between GPs was similar to that found in studies of referral patterns, and the need for further research into the referral process remains. This research will be particularly important for mental health services, where recent developments in community services have brought the current roles of psychiatrists and GPs under considerable scrutiny (Shepherd, 1982; Wilkinson, 1989).

The link between list size and incidence which has emerged in this analysis takes on a special significance because of the current debate over the relationship of list size to the quality of care in general practice. This debate has been fuelled by the high profile given to medical audit in the White Paper "Working for Patients" (White Paper, 1989), which has raised conflicting views on measures of quality and efficiency in general practice. It has been suggested that the changes put forward in the White Paper will "shift the mix of financial and professional incentives" (Howie et al, 1989) towards longer list sizes and shorter consultation times. The influence of list size on referral to psychiatric care requires further investigation to assess how the predicted changes may influence the pattern of care received by the mentally ill in general practice. The results from this analysis suggest that people with certain psychosocial problems, such as anxiety disorders or drug dependencies, will become increasingly 'invisible'.

References
Blacker C V R, Clare A W, 1987, "Depressive disorder in primary care" *British Journal of Psychiatry* **150** 737–751
Brown G W, Harris T, 1978 *Social Origins of Depression* (Tavistock Publications, Andover, Hants)
Brown P J B, Batey P W J, 1987, "A national classification of 1981 census enumeration districts: the derivation of super profile area types", area classification information note 1, Centre for Urban Studies, University of Liverpool, PO Box 147, Liverpool L69 3BX
Corney R H, 1984, "The effectiveness of attached social workers in the management of depressed female patients in general practice" *Psychological Medicine* **6** (supplement)
Davenport S, Goldberg D, Millard T, 1987, "How psychiatric disorders are missed during medical consultations" *Lancet* **ii** 439–441
Dowie R, 1983, "General practitioners and consultants: a study of out-patient referrals" (King Edward's Hospital Fund for London, London)
Fitzpatrick R, Hinton J, Newman S, Scambler G, Thompson J, 1984 *The Experience of Illness* (Tavistock Publications, Andover, Hants)
Freeling P, Rao B M, Paykel E S, Sireling L I, Burton R H, 1985, "Unrecognised depression in general practice" *British Medical Journal* **290** 1880–1883
Ginnsberg G, Marks I, Waters H, 1984, "Cost–benefit analysis of a controlled trial of nurse therapy for neuroses in primary care" *Psychological Medicine* **14** 683–690
Goldberg D P, Blackwell B, 1970, "Psychiatric illness in general practice—a detailed study using a new method of case identification" *British Medical Journal* **261** 439–443
Goldberg D P, Huxley P, 1980 *Mental Illness in the Community* (Tavistock Publications, Andover, Hants)
Goldberg D P, Steele J, Smith C, Spivey L, 1980, "Training family practice residents to recognise psychiatric disturbances", final report, number ADAMHA 278-78-003 (DB), Department of Psychiatry, Biometrics and Family Practice, Medical University of South Carolina, 171 Ashley Avenue, Charleston, SC 29425
Good B J, 1977, "The heart of what's the matter" *Culture, Medicine and Psychiatry* **1**(1) 25–58

Hagnell O, 1966 *A Prospective Study of the Incidence of Mental Disorder* (Svenska Bokforlaget Bonniers, Stockholm)

HCSSSC, 1985, "Community care", second report, House of Commons Social Services Select Committee (HMSO, London)

Howie J R G, Porter A M D, Forbes J F, 1989, "Quality and the use of time in general practice: widening the discussion" *British Medical Journal* **298** 1008-1010

Hurry J, Tennant C, Bebbington P E, 1980, "The selective factors leading to psychiatric referral" *Acta Psychiatrica Scandinavia* **285** (supplement) 315-324

Jenkins R, Shepherd M, 1983, "Mental illness in general practice", in *Mental Illness: Changes and Trends* Ed. P Bean (John Wiley, Chichester, Sussex) pp 132-138

Marks J, Goldberg D, Hillier V F, 1979, "Determinants of the ability of general practitioners to detect psychiatric illness" *Psychological Medicine* **9** 337-353

Mechanic D, 1982, "The epidemiology of illness behaviour and its relation to physical and psychosocial stress", in *Symptoms, Illness Behaviour and Help-seeking* Ed. D Mechanic (Prodist, New York) pp 81-84

Munk-Jorgensen P, 1986, "General practitioners' selection of patients for treatment in community psychiatric services" *Psychological Medicine* **16** 611-619

Nutter R D, Thomas R W, 1990, "An analysis of psychiatric patient attributes in Salford using categorical data models" *Social Science and Medicine* **30** 83-94

Parkin D, 1979, "Distance as an influence on demand in general practice" *Epidemiology and Community Health* **33** 96-99

Phillips D R, 1981 *Contemporary Issues in the Geography of Health Care* (Geo Books, Norwich)

Scobie S, 1989 *The Use of Psychiatric Services in Salford 1970-72 and 1980-82* unpublished PhD thesis, School of Geography, University of Manchester, Manchester M13 9PL

Shaw G, Wheeler D, 1985 *Statistical Techniques in Geographical Analysis* (John Wiley, Chichester, Sussex)

Shepherd M, 1982, "Who should treat mental disorders?" *Lancet* i 1173-1175

Shepherd M, Cooper B, Brown A C, Kalton G W, 1966 *Psychiatric Illness in General Practice* (Oxford University Press, Oxford)

Smith C J, Giggs J A (Eds), 1988 *Location and Stigma: Contemporary Perspectives on Mental Health and Mental Health Care* (Unwin Hyman, London)

Tryer P, 1985, "Psychiatric clinics in general practice" *British Journal of Psychiatry* **145** 9-14

Tryer P, Turner R, Johnson A L, 1989, "Integrated hospital and community psychiatric services and use of in-patient beds" *British Medical Journal* **289** 298-300

Weissman M M, Myers J K, 1978, "Rates and risk of depressive symptoms in a US urban community" *Acta Psychiatrica Scandinavia* **57**(3) 219-231

Whitehouse C R, 1987, "A survey of the management of psychosocial illness in general practice in Manchester" *Journal of the Royal College of General Practitioners* **37** 112-115

White Paper, 1989, "Working for patients" (HMSO, London)

Wilkin D, Metcalfe D H H, 1984, "List size and patient contact in general medical practice" *British Medical Journal* **289** 1501-1505

Wilkin D, Smith A G, 1987, "Variation in general practitioners' referral rates to consultants" *Journal of the Royal College of General Practitioners* **37** 350-353

Wilkin D, Hallan L, Leavey R, Metcalfe D H H, 1987 *Anatomy of Urban General Practice* (Tavistock Publications, Andover, Hants)

Wilkinson G, 1989, "Referrals from GPs to psychiatrists and paramedical mental health professionals" *British Journal of Psychiatry* **154** 72–76

Williams P, Balestrieri M, 1989, "Psychiatric clinics in general practice: do they reduce admissions?" *British Journal of Psychiatry* **154** 67–71

Wilson S, Wilson K, 1985, "Close encounters in general practice" *British Journal of Psychiatry* **146** 277–281

Wooff K, Goldberg D P, 1988, "Further observations on the practice of community care in Salford" *British Journal of Psychiatry* **153** 30–37

Wooff K, Freeman H L, Fryers T, 1983, "Psychiatric service use in Salford" *British Journal of Psychiatry* **142** 588–597

Wooff K, Goldberg D P, Fryers T, 1986, "Patients in receipt of community psychiatric nursing care in Salford 1976–1982" *Psychological Medicine* **16** 407–414

Wooff K, Goldberg D P, Fryers T, 1988, "The practice of community care in Salford" *British Journal of Psychiatry* **153** 30–37

Drug Abuse and Urban Ecological Structure: The Nottingham Case

J A GIGGS
University of Nottingham

1 Introduction
Since prehistoric times man has devised and used certain substances (notably alcohol, tobacco, caffeine, cannabis, opioids, and cocaine) to modify mood or behaviour for a variety of purposes: as part of magic or religious rituals, for medical or purely recreational reasons (see Reed, 1980, page 219). There are substantial societal, subcultural, and temporal variations in attitudes towards specific drugs and the particular contexts in which they are used. However, the majority of drug users in almost every society participate only intermittently, moderately, and in socially approved and prescribed settings. In contrast, a minority uses drugs in socially unacceptable ways (for example, illegally or in excessive quantities, either episodically or for protracted periods) (see Davies and Walsh, 1983; Reed, 1980, page 219; Smith and Hanham, 1982).

There is ample evidence that the more or less regular use of many drugs affects the central nervous system and induces behavioural changes. This voluntary and sustained use of drugs (often for as little as a month) is categorised as pathological substance abuse and results in impaired occupational functioning and social relations. Indeed, such behaviour has been categorised as mental disorder (see APA, 1980, page 163), and classified specifically as *volitional* disorder (see Mulé, 1981). Protracted substance abuse can lead in turn to progressively more severe forms of illness, namely substance *dependence* (that is, a state requiring physiological dependence and habitual behaviour directed towards acquisition of the drugs), and substance-induced organic mental disorders (that is, organic brain syndromes). Ultimately, pathological drug use can result in premature death. Thus, the American Psychiatric Association (APA, 1980, page 172) states that:

"In the United States, in this century, persons with Opioid Dependence have a high death rate (approximately 10 per 1,000) because of the physical complications of the disorder and a lifestyle often associated with violence."

In the United Kingdom the nonmedical use of many drugs (especially opiates) has traditionally been relatively insignificant compared with the experience of the USA. West and Cohen (1985, page 129) attribute the more favourable British experience to the fact that in 1920 Parliament passed the Dangerous Drugs Act, restricting opiate supply to professional physicians. More importantly, the Act permitted them to prescribe opiates to addicted patients (that is, to treat their addiction as a medical condition rather than a criminal activity). Between 1935 and 1951 the numbers of registered opiate addicts fell from 700 to 301. By 1960 only 15 new cases were reported in Britain (see West and Cohen, 1985, page 129). Thereafter the numbers of new registered narcotic drug addicts began to increase throughout the 1960s and 1970s, primarily as a result of the novel 'recreational' use of illegal drugs by young people (see Edwards and Busch, 1981). During the past decade, however, the United Kingdom has, apparently, experienced an 'epidemic' of drug taking, with the numbers of notified new narcotic drug addicts rising from 984 in 1976, to 6409 in 1985 (see Home Office, 1989). These figures undoubtedly represent only a fraction of the actual numbers engaged in narcotic drug abuse. Unfortunately it is not possible to obtain a precise figure for the true prevalence because there are now many addicts who are not registered with physicians (see Mott, 1986). In 1988 12 977 addicts were recorded as receiving notifiable drugs in treatment of addiction. However, research commissioned by the DHSS (1982) suggests that the total number of opioid addicts in the United Kingdom may be at least 5 times the number notified. Such estimates need to be treated with caution. Mott (1986) and Plant (1989) have noted that there are no routine national surveys of drug use in Britain, unlike in the USA and Canada. Instead, intermittent sample studies of specific sections of the British population and a few detailed local prevalence studies have identified marked social, spatial, and temporal variations in the prevalence of drug abuse (see Parker et al, 1987; Plant, 1989).

Furthermore, some researchers have argued that the rising prevalence rates of drug abuse and other social and health problems do not in fact represent 'real' increases, but are deliberately inflated for political, economic, and professional reasons. MacGregor (1989) has asserted that this process of inflating prevalence rates to epidemic proportions has tended to generate a variety of highly publicised and emotionally charged 'moral panics'.

Despite the profound difficulties involved in quantifying accurately the scale of the problem, narcotic drug abuse does, justifiably, cause widespread concern. Part of this concern can be attributed to the fact that the majority of the victims become addicted when they are young and entering what should be the most productive stages of their lives. In 1985 23.9% of the registered new addicts in the United Kingdom were aged under 20 years, and 76.8% were aged under 30 years (see Home Office, 1989). In addition, many drug abusers engage in criminal activities as a direct consequence of their addiction. The research on drug taking and crime in Britain has been reviewed comprehensively by Mott (1981) and Bean et al (1987). Last, there is substantial evidence that drug abuse impairs health and reduces life expectancy (see Plant, 1989; Smith and Hanham, 1982; West and Cohen, 1985). During the 1980s the health-related risks of narcotic drug abuse have multiplied with the emergence and global spread of the increasing spectrum of human immune deficiency virus (HIV) diseases and their ultimate, fatal stage namely the acquired immune deficiency syndrome (AIDS) (see Mann et al, 1988; Redfield and Burke, 1988). Drug misusers who are infected can transmit HIV by sharing needles, syringes, and other equipment which have become contaminated wih infected blood. In addition, infected misusers can also transmit HIV sexually into the general population. At present there are marked national, regional, and local variations in HIV seroprevalence rates amongst intravenous drug misusers (see DHSS, 1981; Mann et al, 1988). Nevertheless, the virus is known to have spread very rapidly through the drug-injecting community in some cities, notably Edinburgh in the United Kingdom, and New York, Los Angeles, and San Francisco in the USA (see DHSS, 1981). Vigorous preventive measures will need to be taken to stem the projected likely upsurge in the numbers of HIV cases among drug users; the increase also being attributable to sexual transmission and the passing on of the infection to foetuses (see DHSS, 1981; Fineberg, 1988).

2 Locality-based studies of drug abuse in the United Kingdom
Until the mid-1960s there were very few drug addicts in the United Kingdom and the problem was largely confined to London (see Spear, 1969). Thereafter the numbers of new narcotic addicts notified to the Home Office (1989) increased markedly, especially outside London. Consequently, between 1973 and 1987 the share of the total new narcotic addicts in the Metropolitan Police Force area fell (in relative terms) from 57.2% to 35% (see Home Office, 1989). Most of the increase in drug abuse outside Greater London took place in just a few urban areas. Thus Ditton and Speirits (1981) found big increases in heroin use in Greater Glasgow between 1979 and 1981. In their analysis of heroin use throughout the north of England, Pearson et al (1987) identified similar 'epidemic' increases mainly in several towns and cities in Lancashire and Cheshire, notably Manchester, Chester, and within Merseyside.

Since 1987 the Statistics Department of the Home Office (1989) has published data concerning drug addicts for the 216 District Health Authorities (DHAs) in the United Kingdom. The number of new addicts notified during 1987 and 1988 in each DHA were aggregated and the average annual incidence rates per 10000 adults were calculated, using the Office of Population Censuses and Surveys's (OPCS, 1988) and General Register Office's (GRO, 1988) midyear estimates of resident population for 1987. The results of this analysis are shown in figure 1. Of the 200 DHAs in the United Kingdom only 61 had average annual incidence rates in excess of 1 per 10000 persons. Greater London accounted for 21 of these, with the highest rates occurring in central London, peaking at 35.7 per 10000 residents in the Paddington and North Kensington DHA. Outside Greater London a second major cluster (comprising 18 DHAs) was found straddling the neighbouring Mersey and North Western Hospital regions. Here, 5 DHAs had rates in excess of 5 per 10 000 residents, namely Liverpool, South Sefton, Chester, Warrington, and Central Manchester. Outside these 2 major clusters, 22 DHAs (including Nottingham) with rates in the range 1 – 4.9 new addicts per 10 000 residents were scattered widely across the rest of England and central Scotland.

During the 1980s several researchers have sought to determine the prevalence (that is, extent) or incidence (number of new addicts) of narcotic drug use in specific British cities. Thus high rates were identified by

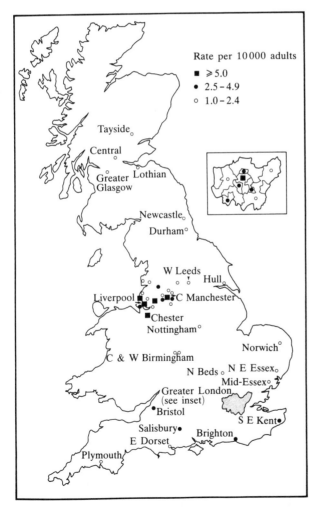

Figure 1. Average annual incidence of notified drug abuse in the United Kingdom, 1987/88.

O'Bryan (1985) and Hartnoll et al (1985b) in London, by Haw (1985) in Greater Glasgow, and by Parker et al (1986; 1987) in Wirral, Merseyside. In contrast, medium to low rates were found by Peveler et al (1988) in Oxford, by Pattison et al (1982) in South Tyneside, and by Levy (1985) in Brighton. These investigations are important because they are not based simply on the official notifications to the Home Office. In every case the researchers have used a range of direct and indirect methods to estimate the prevalence and incidence of various types of drug taking. This important research has been stimulated by the work of the London-based Drug Indicators Project (see Hartnoll et al, 1985a). Thus Parker et al (1986; 1987) adopted the *multiagency* enumeration method of prevalence estimation in their survey of heroin abuse in Wirral, Merseyside. They consulted 10 agencies and identified 1305 heroin users, of whom only 273 had been notified to the Home Office.

Some of these researchers have also been concerned about the spatial manifestations of the drug-abuse problem. Thus Parker et al (1986; 1987) and Pearson et al (1987) mapped the distribution of addicts and discovered high rates among the residents of deprived inner-city neighbourhoods and in some council estates. However, several equally deprived neighbourhoods had either no drug addicts or very few. Pearson et al (1987) attributed this phenomenon to the absence of drug-supply networks in these localities. They also argued that housing-allocation policies which use certain council estates as 'dumping grounds' for difficult tenants contribute to the concentrations of drug abuse and other social problems. Several authors also demonstrate the existence of a major drug-abuse problem in a few prosperous neighbourhoods, though these are located adjacent to neighbourhoods characterised by high levels of heroin abuse and serious social and housing deprivation (see Dorn and South, 1985; Parker et al, 1986; 1987; Pearson et al, 1987).

Although no geographers have yet addressed any aspect of the British drug abuse problem, it is clear that their work in related urban, social, and medical fields makes them eminently fitted to make valuable contributions in this burgeoning field of research. Thus there are strong similarities between the questions being addressed and the research strategies employed by drug abuse epidemiologists and those found in recent geographical investigations of health, and of crime, delinquency, and other urban social problems (see Evans and Herbert, 1989; Herbert, 1982; Jones and Moon, 1987; Smith and Giggs, 1988; Winchester and White, 1988).

3 Drug abuse in Greater Nottingham
The findings presented here constitute part of a broader study of drug taking in Nottingham and the links with crime (see Bean et al, 1987). The study focused on nonmedical users of class A drugs, namely the opiates, synthetic opiates (primarily physeptone and methadone), LSD,

and injected amphetamines. Following Hartnoll et al (1985a), we used the *multienumeration* method to identify cases for the year ending 31 March 1986. The agencies involved were: the Home Office, the Trent Region Alcohol and Drug Dependency Unit (which is located in Nottingham), the local district general and psychiatric hospitals, the 2 Nottingham courts, the probation service, the social services, and the police. Interviewed users were also asked to name other drug addicts known to them. This 'snowball' technique identified 26 persons not known to any of the above agencies. The survey revealed that 170 drug users were living in the Greater Nottingham area. Only 74 of these active drug users were listed on the Home Office Notified Addicts Index. Thus the Home Office Index included 43.5% of the addicts found in Nottingham, compared with only 20.9% of those found in Wirral District by Parker et al (1987).

4 Nottingham's ecological structure
In their efforts to study and explain drug misuse several British epidemiologists (notably Parker et al, 1987; Pearson et al, 1987) have analysed the relationships between the spatial patterning of drug misuse and the social and environmental attributes of the localities in which it is most prevalent. This strategy was first employed by Faris and Dunham (1939) in their seminal study of the ecology of mental disorders (including drug addiction) in Chicago during the 1920s and early 1930s. Their example has since been emulated and refined in many spatial studies of mental and physical illnesses, crime and delinquency, and other social problems (see Herbert, 1982; Herbert and Smith, 1989; Jones and Moon, 1987; Smith and Giggs, 1988).

Given these substantial methodological and empirical precedents *and* the relative dearth of empirical examples with respect to the ecology of drug misuse, it was considered appropriate to analyse the ways in which drug misuse in Greater Nottingham is related to the ecological structure of the area. Accordingly, 2 multivariate statistical methods, namely principal components analysis and cluster analysis, were employed to identify the ecological structure of the study area. A total of 40 appropriate variables were selected as a data set (table 1). Variables 1–36 were derived from the 1982 small area tabulations of the population census (OPCS, 1982) and variables 37–40 were obtained from Nottinghamshire County Council's Planning Department's surveys of disadvantage in the county (NCC, 1983; 1984).

In the principal components analysis, 5 components with eigenvalues exceeding unity were identified. They accounted for 78.0% of the total variance in the data set. Using the varimax rotation (see table 1), we interpret component 1 as a dimension of social and material resources, with the 'haves' identified by the variables with positive loadings and the 'have nots' by variables with negative loadings. Component 2 is also bipolar in character and is labelled as an axis between status/familism and urbanism. Component 3 is primarily a life-cycle construct, and component 4 is an axis between housing tenure and economic participation.

Table 1. Component loadings.

Variables	Component				
	1	2	3	4	5
1 0-15 years (children)	–	0.549	-0.403	–	0.561
2 16-59 (adults at risk)	0.432	–	-0.640	–	–
3 65 and over	–	–	0.764	–	–
4 Single adults	-0.521	-0.654	–	–	–
5 Two adults	-0.811	–	–	–	–
6 Established families	0.579	0.612	–	–	–
7 Large families	-0.837	–	–	–	–
8 Lone parent families	-0.889	–	–	–	–
9 Single pensioner	-0.503	–	0.743	–	–
10 Economically active women	0.695	–	–	-0.558	–
11 Unemployed adults	-0.992	–	–	–	–
12 Unemployed youths	-0.867	–	–	–	–
13 Sick workers	-0.836	–	–	–	–
14 Agricultural workers	–	–	–	0.479	0.487
15 Energy workers	–	0.736	–	0.435	–
16 Manufacturing workers	–	–	–	-0.556	–
17 Services workers	–	-0.804	–	–	–
18 Professional, managerial	0.742	-0.500	–	–	–
19 Other nonmanual	0.530	-0.632	–	–	–
20 Skilled	–	0.828	–	–	–
21 Semiskilled	-0.654	0.414	–	–	–
22 Unskilled	-0.763	–	–	–	–
23 Students aged 16 or more	0.647	-0.586	–	–	–
24 No car	-0.964	–	–	–	–
25 2 or more cars	0.816	–	–	–	0.408
26 NCWP-born	-0.528	-0.499	–	–	–
27 Irish-born	-0.591	-0.547	–	–	–
28 European-born	–	-0.689	–	–	–
29 Movers, 1980/81	-0.418	-0.535	–	–	–
30 Owner-occupiers	0.835	–	–	–	–
31 Council tenants	-0.706	–	–	–	–
32 Rented unfurnished	–	–	–	0.743	–
33 Rented furnished	–	-0.645	-0.528	–	–
34 Overcrowding	-0.751	–	–	–	–
35 Large dwellings	0.544	-0.591	–	–	–
36 Shared amenities	-0.491	–	–	0.521	–
37 Free school meals	-0.895	–	–	–	–
38 Children at risk	-0.780	–	–	–	–
39 Juvenile crime	-0.796	–	–	–	–
40 Adult crime	-0.554	–	–	–	–
Percentage total variance	39.4	17.8	8.4	7.2	5.2

– Loading less than 0.400.
Note: NCWP New Commonwealth and Pakistan.

Component 5 has medium loadings on only 3 variables but collectively these identified new youthful suburban estates. These 5 dimensions are broadly comparable with those produced by Davies (1984) in his comprehensive analysis of social dimensionality in British cities.

The scores for the 105 zones on the components were then grouped, using the nonhierarchical clustering algorithm described by Mather (1976). This analysis produced an 'optimal' solution of 14 groups of zones. The average scores for these groups are given in table 2. Here the groups have been presented in 4 sets, differentiated primarily by attributes of location, housing tenure, and status (see figure 2). The first set includes groups 1–4 and is labelled *inner-city, mixed tenure*. Group 1 is described as a *low-status* and *transient* type, having very poor social and material resources (component 1) and strong urbanism characteristics (component 2). It includes Nottingham's CBD. Group 2 is labelled low-status and represents most of the city's surviving tracts of nineteenth-century artisan terraced housing. Group 3 comprises 2 contiguous zones located northwest of the city centre, and is a mixture of nineteenth-century terraced housing and a variety of post-1960s council housing (mainly deck-access flats and link housing). Group 4 is described as high-status and transient. It consists of just 3 areas, one on the west side of the city centre (the Park), the other two 3 km north of the city centre (Mapperley Park and Sherwood). Since the mid-nineteenth century, Mapperley Park and the Park have been Nottingham's most prestigious residential areas. Since the mid-1970s they have both been designated

Table 2. Group means for component scores, 1981.

Characteristics of 14 clusters	Component				
	1	2	3	4	5
Inner-city, mixed tenure					
1 Low-status, transient	−1.82	−2.48	−3.33	0.44	−0.30
2 Low-status	−1.22	−0.76	−0.31	0.28	−0.14
3 Low-status with renewal	−3.40	−1.80	−2.83	−0.53	2.94
4 High-status, transient	+1.50	−2.48	−1.56	0.32	−1.43
Older suburbs, mixed tenure, middle status					
5 Postfamily	−0.26	−0.34	1.35	0.60	1.22
6 Established and postfamily	0.29	0.01	0.19	−0.77	−0.86
Low-status, council tenure					
7 Established family, new housing	−2.29	0.05	0.57	−0.70	1.87
8 Established and postfamily	−1.06	0.15	1.44	−1.17	0.03
9 Young and established families	−0.32	0.67	−0.24	−1.82	−0.21
10 As 9, new housing	−0.69	0.49	−0.63	−1.45	1.02
Middle-status to high-status, owner-occupied tenure					
11 Ageing families	0.67	−1.32	1.47	0.28	−0.20
12 Young and established families	1.15	−0.11	−0.49	−1.11	−0.46
13 Established families	1.14	0.99	0.11	−0.59	0.26
14 As 12, new housing	1.10	0.66	−1.63	−1.99	0.11

as conservation areas by Nottingham City Council. The third area in
this group lies south of the city, in West Bridgford.

Groups 5 and 6 constitute the second set. They are collectively
labelled as older suburbs, mixed tenure, and middle-status (table 2). In
housing terms they represent the oldest suburbs in the study area; a
mixture of both Edwardian and interwar housing estates. These fringe
the western and northern margins of nineteenth-century Nottingham, that
is, groups 1–4 (figure 2) and especially the cores of 4 of the 5 satellite
towns surrounding the city. Group 5 zones have very high proportions
of elderly persons and are labelled as postfamily. In contrast, group 6
zones are described as established and postfamily.

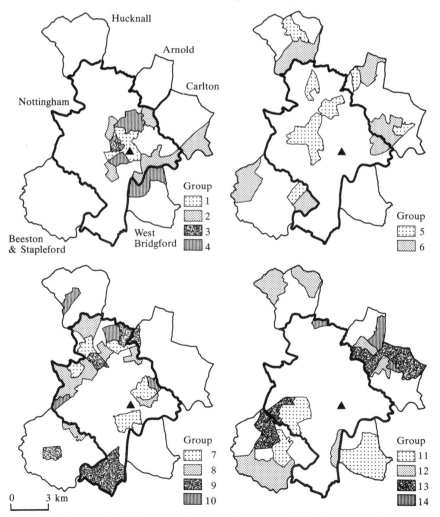

Figure 2. Greater Nottingham and its social areas in 1981. Note: ▲ CBD.

Groups 7-10 are council estates (table 2). In 1981 the zones in these 4 groups housed more than a third of the population of Greater Nottingham. The existence of 4 council-housing groups attests to the size and diversity of this large segment of population and housing stock in the area. Group 7 is labelled established family, new housing. It has the second lowest score for social and material resources (component 1, table 1) and its member zones comprise both the 2 inner-city comprehensive redevelopment zones (that is, St Ann's and the Meadows) and 3 estates with substantial post-1970 extensions located in the north of Nottingham (figure 2). Group 3 is characterised as established and postfamily and has high proportions of elderly persons and economically active women. The estates in this group were built mainly during the 1950s and 1960s. Group 9 estates (young and established families) were also built during this period but are distinguished from group 8 by virtue of having received large numbers of young families from the slum-clearance zones in the inner city during the 1970s (see Brown, 1989). Group 9 zones identify suburban post-1976 council estates, built to house the populations of the inner-city slum-clearance areas.

The fourth set comprises 4 groups and is collectively labelled middle-status to high-status, owner-occupied tenure (table 2). They are the affluent interwar and postwar suburbs of Greater Nottingham (figure 2). Given the fact that Nottingham City Council has, since the 1920s, purchased most of the available land within the city limits for building council housing, private-housing developers have been obliged to concentrate their activities in the neighbouring satellite towns (see Brown, 1989; Thomas, 1971). Thus most of the zones in these groups are located outside the city itself (figure 2). Table 2 reveals that groups 11-14 are differentiated primarily in terms of age and family attributes. However, group 13, represented by just 3 zones, picks out the only substantial areas of owner-occupied housing built in the area between 1970 and 1981.

5 The spatial patterning of Nottingham's drug abusers
Of the 170 active drug abusers identified as living in Greater Nottingham 7 had no fixed abode and therefore could not be mapped. Figure 3 shows the residential distribution of the remaining 163 cases, differentiated by sex and 3 major categories of drug use. The results are striking. Of the 163 drug users 119 (73.0%) lived in the city itself and only 44 lived in the 5 contiguous suburbs. Furthermore, most of the drug takers were clustered mainly in the city's inner residential areas, fringing the city centre. Thus 62.6% of all drug takers lived within 4 km of the city centre. However, as table 3 shows, there are interesting variations in the zonal distributions of the three major categories of drug user. Figure 3 also reveals that, in addition to the substantial inner-city concentration of drug users, there are several large secondary groups. Specifically there

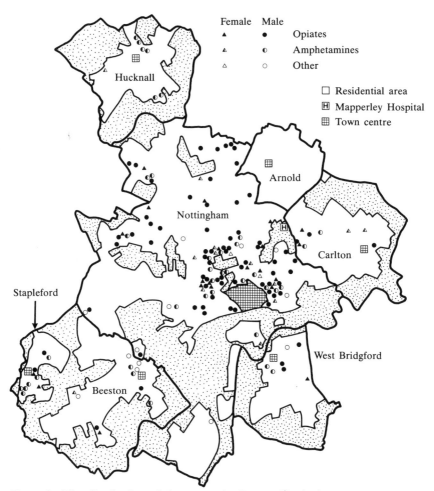

Figure 3. The distribution of drug users in Greater Nottingham, 1985/86.

Table 3. Zonal distribution of drug takers in Greater Nottingham.

Zones[a] (km)	All users		Opioid users		Other drug[b] users	
	number	percent	number	percent	number	percent
0–2	68	41.7	44	44.9	24	36.9
2–4	34	20.9	22	22.4	12	18.5
4–6	36	22.1	22	22.4	14	21.5
6–8	9	5.5	6	6.1	3	4.6
8–10	11	6.7	4	4.1	7	10.8
10–12	5	3.1	0	0.0	5	7.7
Total	163	100.0	98	100.0	65	100.0

[a] Concentric rings around Nottingham city centre.
[b] Includes amphetamines, hallucinogens, and so on.

are 3 clusters located in the northwestern and western suburbs of Nottingham, and 5 other clusters, chiefly fringing the small suburban town centres of Hucknall, West Bridgford, Beeston, and Stapleford. In Carlton, however, most of the drug users lived close to Mapperley Psychiatric Hospital rather than Carlton town centre. Arnold is an atypical suburb, for no drug users were identified as living there.

Further insights into the distribution of Nottingham's drug abusers can be gained by calculating and mapping prevalence rates per capita for appropriate subareas. However, Choynowski (1959) has suggested that *probability* mapping is a superior technique, particularly when the number of events (in this case, drug addicts) is comparatively small. The spatial variation in the number of drug abusers occurring in Greater Nottingham was therefore tested by means of the Poisson probability formula (see Norcliffe, 1977). This test was applied to the raw data, namely the 'at risk' population (that is, persons aged 16 years and over) and the numbers of drug users living in the 14 groups of zones identified in table 2 and figure 2. The analysis included total drug users and 2 subgroups, 'opioid users' and 'users of all other drugs'. The results are given in table 4. There were significantly high numbers of cases for all these sets of drug abusers in just 2 of the 14 groups, namely groups 1 and 7. In contrast the neighbourhoods comprising group 3 had significantly large numbers only in the categories of all users and opioid users. These 3 groups are primarily inner-city neighbourhoods (figure 2) and have the worst social

Table 4. Probability levels for drug abuse in Greater Nottingham.

Groups	All users	Opioid users	Other drug users
Inner-city, mixed tenure			
1 Low-status, transient	+ +	+ +	+ +
2 Low-status			
3 Low-status with renewal	+ +	+ +	
4 High-status, transient	+		+
Older suburbs, mixed tenure, middle-status			
5 Postfamily	- -	-	-
6 Established and postfamily		-	
Low-status, council tenure			
7 Established family, new housing	+ +	+ +	+
8 Established and postfamily			
9 Young and established families	- -	-	-
10 As 9, new housing			
Middle-status to high-status, owner-occupied tenure			
11 Ageing families			
12 Young and established families	- -	-	-
13 Established families	-	-	
14 As 12, new housing	-	-	

+ + Probability levels greater than 0.01   + Probability levels greater than 0.05
- - Probability levels less than 0.01   - Probability levels less than 0.05

and material resources in Greater Nottingham (see component 1 scores in table 2). A fourth group (group 4) has a moderately significant excess of cases in the categories of 'all users' and 'other drug users'. This is the highest-status set of zones in Greater Nottingham (component 1, table 2). However, figure 2 shows that they are located in the inner city, adjacent to the 'high-risk' low-status neighbourhoods (that is, groups 1, 3, and 7). In addition, all 4 high-risk groups of zones are characterised by high rates of population turnover, as indexed by the residential mobility variable, by slum clearance and redevelopment in the inner city (chiefly affecting zones in groups 3 and 7), and by the building of new houses (particularly important in groups 3, 4, and 7).

In contrast, the areas with significantly *low* numbers of drug abusers are all found in the middle and outer suburbs of Greater Nottingham. Here, 6 groups have low numbers for 1 or more of the 3 categories of drug users (table 4). These include groups 5 and 6—the middle-status older suburbs—3 of the 4 middle-status to high-status owner-occupied suburb groups (that is, groups 12, 13, and 14), and 1 of the 4 low-status, council-tenure sets (that is, group 9).

These findings suggest that, in broad terms, there is a significant concentration of drug abusers in Greater Nottingham's lower-status, inner-city neighbourhoods. However, there are interesting and important exceptions to this generalisation. Thus the high-status inner-city group 4 zones have significantly high numbers for 2 categories of drug users whereas the low-status group 2 zones do not have significantly more drug users than might be expected by chance. The group 2 zones are located around the outer fringes of the high concentrations of drug users (figures 2 and 3) and probably have no resident drug suppliers. In the low-status suburban council estates, in contrast, there are non-significant numbers of drug users in groups 8 and 10, and significantly low numbers of users in group 9. It is only in the 3 northern outliers of group 7 that significantly high numbers of drug users are found. These areas received large numbers of residents during the redevelopment of the slums in St Ann's and there is some evidence that the city housing department used them as 'dumping grounds' for problem families (see NCC, 1983; 1984; Simpson, 1981).

The evidence presented here therefore appears to support the findings of Parker et al (1986; 1987) and Pearson et al (1987). High rates of drug abuse are found in localities where there are effective drug-supply networks. These are primarily concentrated in neighbourhoods characterised by high levels of social and material deprivation. However, high rates of drug abuse are often found in high-status neighbourhoods where these are located adjacent to low-status areas possessing suppliers and large numbers of drug abusers. In contrast, there are low-status neighbourhoods in both inner-city and suburban locations which lack drug suppliers and significant numbers of users. In addition, in some inner-city and suburban low-status council estates, it would appear that the operation of selective 'dumping' policies by local housing officers has resulted in the unwitting creation of localised concentrations of drug-supply and drug-abuse problems.

6 Links between drug abuse and ecological structure

Researchers into the spatial ecology of drug abuse have tried to identify key correlates of rates of incidence of drug abusers and to use these as bases of explanation (see Parker et al, 1987; Pearson et al, 1987). However, they argue that emphasis should be placed on understanding the general conditions under which drug abuse is precipitated rather than simply trying to identify causes, as these are known to be complex (see Home Office, 1984). Given that the few existing studies have demonstrated the complexity of the relationships between drug abuse and a range of social and environmental variables, the present analysis was based upon the 3 drug-abuse variables (table 4) and the 5 sets of component scores for the 14 groups of zones (table 2). In the present investigation, stepwise regression was employed to measure the relationships between drug abuse and the social–environmental attributes represented by these 5 sets of area traits. A further advantage of using component scores as input is that this procedure helps to overcome the multicollinearity problem.

Table 5 provides summary descriptions of the 3 stepwise regression analyses. In all 3 cases only 2 components were included as a result of the default value listed in the analyses ($T = 0.05$). The results show that component 1—(poor) social and material resources—had the strongest associations with areas of residence of all drug users and of opioid drug users. For the other drug users, component 1 was the second independent variable to enter the equation. Component 3—life-cycle (specifically the 15–59 year olds and rented furnished tenure)—was the second most important construct in the explanation of variation in the distribution of all drug users and opioid drug users. In the equation for other drug users, component 2—status/familism and urbanism—emerged as the first and most significant explanatory variable (see table 1).

Table 5. Stepwise regression results.

Variable	Components	Adjusted R^2
All drug users	1 Social and material resources	0.646[*]
	3 Life-cycle (young[a], rented furnished)	0.810[*]
Opioid drug users	1 Social and material resources	0.621[*]
	3 Life-cycle (young[a], rented furnished)	0.754[*]
Other drug users	2 Status/familism and urbanism	0.540[*]
	1 Social and material resources	0.640[*]

[*] F-values significant at the 0.01 level. [a] Aged 15–59 years old.

7 Demographic, social, and behavioural attributes of Nottingham's drug abusers

During the course of the survey of the drug-abuse problem in Greater Nottingham a considerable amount of information was obtained from the respondents via a detailed questionnaire (see Bean et al, 1987). From these data, an important complement to the aggregate analyses presented above was provided. The survey revealed that Nottingham's drug abusers are predominantly male (78.2% of all drug users, 73.5% of all opioid drug users, 86.0% of all other drug users). They are also mainly Caucasian (91.8%).

The analysis of drug users by age-groups (table 6) provides further important insights. None of the known drug users in Greater Nottingham were under 16 years of age and only 5 (3.0%) were aged 45 years or more. For two groups (that is, total users and opioid users) the highest rates were recorded for persons in the 25–34 years age bracket. For 'other drug users', the highest rate was found among 16–24 year olds. There are substantial age-group variations between the different groups of drug users (table 6). Thus 23.5% of all the drug users were aged 16–24 years, compared with 42.6% of the 'other drug users'. These findings differ markedly from those found in other recent surveys, notably that of Wirral by Parker et al (1987). In Wirral the annual prevalence rate of opioid abuse during 1984/85 was 18.2 per 1000 people among persons aged 16–24, compared with only 0.16 per 1000 people in Nottingham during 1985/86. Moreover, the 16–24 year olds accounted for 75% of all the opioid abusers in Wirral, compared with only 10.8% in Nottingham.

Only 17% of Nottingham's drug users were married and living with their spouses. A further 37% were cohabiting. A total of 40% of the drug users lived in households which contained children: 31% lived with their own children, 6% lived with children of relatives, and 4% lived with children of friends. Only 25% of all users lived alone.

Table 6. The age distribution of known, problem, drug users in Greater Nottingham, 1985/86.

Age	Population	All drug users			Opioid users			Other drug users		
		no.	rate	%	no.	rate	%	no.	rate	%
16–24	70147	40	0.57	23.5	11	0.16	10.8	29	0.41	42.6
25–34	66350	81	1.22	47.6	57	0.86	55.9	24	0.36	35.3
35–44	53838	44	0.82	25.9	32	0.59	31.4	12	0.22	17.6
⩾45	185177	5	0.03	2.9	2	0.01	2.0	3	0.02	4.4
Total	375512	170	0.45	100.0	102	0.27	100.0	68	0.18	100.0

Note: Rate is the number of cases per 1000 residents; percent is the number of cases as a percent of the column total.

Only 11% of the drug users were employed at the time of interview. Manual occupations accounted for 5.9%, skilled occupations for 1.2%, 2.4% were self-employed, and 1.2% (2 persons) were professionals. Of the unemployed drug users 80% had been so for over 12 months. In this sense, data on social class was largely meaningless.

A total of 20% of the drug abusers claimed that they had first obtained drugs from their spouse, cohabitee, or boyfriend or girlfriend. A further 47% had first obtained drugs from a close friend or acquaintance. Over three quarters (77%) had first used cannabis or amphetamines, and only 2.4% had first used opioids. However, at the time of interview, 60% were using opioids. Most of the drug abusers were heavily engaged in drug taking, with 81% taking drugs every day and only 3.5% using drugs one day a week or less.

At the time of interview 69% of the opioid drug users were in treatment at the Trent Regional Drug Addiction Unit, based at Mapperley Hospital. In contrast, only 6% of the 'other drug' users were in treatment. This disparity can be attributed to the fact that among Nottingham's drug users only the opioid users are viewed as being 'drug addicts'. It is further perceived that the Addiction Unit was only for drug addicts (that is, opioid users). Consequently the majority of the nonopioid users obtain their supplies through the illicit system, whereas the opioid drug users exploit both the licit (that is, Addiction Unit prescriptions) and illicit supply systems. Given their very limited financial resources, crime is a way of life for Nottingham's drug users, primarily in order to 'feed the habit'. Of the 170 drug users 93% admitted to having at least one conviction and the rest had all engaged in nonreported criminal activity. Self-report information revealed that many drug abusers were themselves the victims of crime: 18% claimed to have been physically attacked, and 46% had been victims of household crimes (22% had been robbed or burgled at least twice). A total of 55% of drug users said they had been the victims of crimes which involved drugs and 48% said they knew the offender, though only 15.7% said that they had reported the crimes. It is evident, therefore, that crime is an integral part of their lives.

Many of the drug abusers are residentially mobile. This would appear to be largely a function of their precarious, vulnerable, and often criminogenic life-style. Many of the drug abusers appeared to be the typical 'itinerant junkies' moving around the country. Thus 14.5% of the cohort had lived in Nottingham for less than 12 months prior to interview. Moreover, all of these in-migrants had settled in the low-status areas located in central Nottingham and shown in figure 5. In addition, a further 32.4% (that is, 55 users) were known to have left the area after the first interview. Of these out-migrants 91% had lived in low-status areas depicted in figure 5. All the out-migrants were opioid drug users and it is presumed that the major reason for their exodus was the discovery that the sole source of licit drug supply in Greater

Nottingham is the Addiction Unit. Moreover, a compulsory condition of supply there is that addicts must enrol in the detoxification programme.

Among the remaining 115 users, 7 claimed to have had no permanent abode in the area in the previous 12 months. In addition, 28 users had changed address at least once within Greater Nottingham in the 12 months

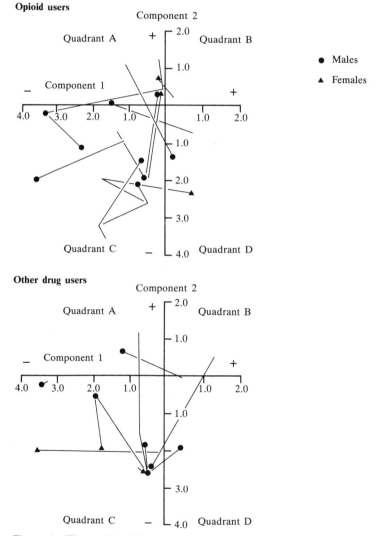

Figure 4. The residential moves of drug users in the social space of Greater Nottingham.

Note: *Component 1* positive extreme good social and material resources; negative extreme poor social and material resources.

Component 2 positive extreme familism and suburbs; negative extreme urbanism and inner city.

prior to interview. Of these moves, 6 had been essentially local (that is, within the same zone—see figure 5). However, most of the others were quite long moves through both the social and the geographical space of the area (see figures 4 and 5). Of these 28 movers, 16 used opioids, and 12 used other drugs. For both groups of users most of the moves took place within the lowest-status areas, namely quadrant C in figure 4 and in the quintile of zones with the lowest scores (that is, the worst social and material resources) on component 1, depicted in figure 5. Of the entire cohort of drug users, therefore, only 32.5% had not changed address during the previous 12 months. The rate of residential mobility among drug abusers would therefore seem to be even higher than that found for other categories of mental disorder (see Giggs, 1984; Giggs and Cooper, 1986).

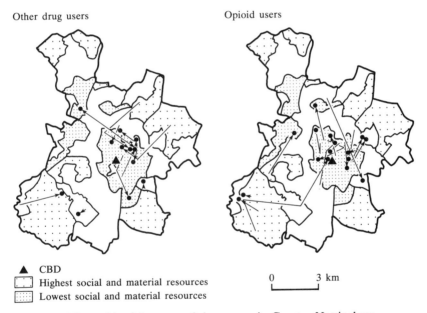

Other drug users

Opioid users

▲ CBD
Highest social and material resources
Lowest social and material resources

0   3 km

Figure 5. The residential moves of drug users in Greater Nottingham.

8 Conclusions

Data published by the Home Office (1989) suggest that there has been a substantial increase in narcotic drug abuse in the United Kingdom since the mid-1970s. Analysis of the spatial patterning of the incidence of drug abuse within the United Kingdom in 1987/88 shows that this epidemic has been highly localised in its effects, with the greatest concentrations of new cases being found in central London and in 18 DHAs in northwest England (figure 1).

Analyses of the prevalence and incidence of narcotic drug abuse in a handful of localities have revealed that the Home Office statistics under-record the true scale of the problem by between 50% and 80%. In the present study too, it was found that drug users notified to the Home Office represented only 43.5% of those identified by multienumeration methods in Greater Nottingham.

There was evidence of substantial (and statistically significant) spatial variations in the prevalence of drug abuse within Greater Nottingham. The problem was greatest in central city neighbouourhoods, and in several secondary suburban pockets. Stepwise regression analysis of the prevalence rates for 3 sets of drug users and the component scores for a 14-group typology of Nottingham's social areas suggested strong links between levels of drug abuse and poor social and material resources (component 1, table 1), inner-city milieux (that is, component 2, table 1), and the life-cycle and tenure construct (that is, component 3, table 1). The findings of these aggregate (that is, ecological) analyses were generally strongly supported by the demographic, social and behavioural data obtained from the drug users via detailed questionnaires.

These findings are broadly similar to those produced in a few earlier studies, notably those of Parker et al (1987) and Pearson et al (1987). In Nottingham too, it was discovered that the relationship between neighbourhood levels of drug abuse and indicators of socioeconomic and housing deprivation was not a simple one. Complicating factors include: first, local housing-allocation policies which use selected inner-city and suburban council estates as dumping grounds for difficult tenants; second, the absence of drug suppliers in certain deprived neighbourhoods which are socially and environmentally identical to those in which drug abuse is rife; and third, the existence of substantial levels of drug abuse in some high-status neighbourhoods when these are located close to low-status areas possessing large numbers of drug abusers and well-organised drug-supply networks.

Comparison of the findings of this with earlier British studies also reveals important differences. Chief among these are the substantial variations in the interurban rates of drug abuse (figure 1) and in the contrasting demographic, social, and behavioural attributes of drug abusers between cities. These matters certainly merit further investigation, and geographers ought to be involved in this work.

Acknowledgement. The author wishes to thank the Home Office for financing this study of drug abuse in Nottingham.

References

APA, 1980 *Diagnostic and Statistical Manual of Mental Disorders* third edition, American Psychiatric Association, Washington, DC

Bean P, Wilkinson C K, Giggs J A, Whynes D K, 1987, "Drug taking in Nottingham and the links with crime", report to the Home Office Research and Planning Unit; copy available from The Home Office, 50 Queen Anne's Gate, London SW1

Brown P, A, 1989, "The development of Nottingham", in *A New Geography of Nottingham* Eds S Brazier, R Hammond, S R Waterman, P A Brown (Trent Polytechnic, Burton Street, Nottingham NG1 4BU) pp 27–38

Choynowski M, 1959, "Maps based on probabilities" *Journal of the American Statistical Association* **54** 385–388

Davies P, Walsh D, 1983 *Alcohol Problems and Alcohol Control in Europe* (Croom Helm, Andover, Hants)

Davies W K D, 1984 *Factorial Ecology* (Gower, Aldershot, Hants)

DHSS, 1981 *AIDS and Drug Misuse, Part 1: Report by the Advisory Council on the Misuse of Drugs* (Academic Press, London)

DHSS, 1982 *Treatment and Rehabilitation: Report of the Advisory Council on the Misuse of Drugs* (HMSO, London)

Ditton J, Speirits K, 1981, "The rapid increase of heroin addiction in Glasgow during 1981" *Background Papers* available from Department of Sociology, University of Glasgow, Glasgow G12 8QQ

Dorn N, South N, 1985 *Helping Drug Users* (Gower, Aldershot, Hants)

Edwards G, Busch C (Eds), 1981 *Drug Problems in Britain: A Review of Ten Years* (Academic Press, London)

Evans D J, Herbert D T (Eds), 1989 *The Geography of Crime* (Routledge, Chapman and Hall, Andover, Hants)

Faris R E L, Dunham H W, 1939 *Mental Disorders in Urban Areas* (University of Chicago Press, Chicago, IL)

Fineberg H V, 1988, "The social dimensions of AIDS" *Scientific Americann* **259**(4) 106–112

Giggs J A, 1984, "Residential mobility and mental health", in *Mental Health and the Environment* Ed. H L Freeman (Churchill Livingstone, Edinburgh) pp 327–356

Giggs J A, Cooper J, 1986, "Mental disorders and human ecological structure: a case study of schizophrenia and affective psychosis in Nottingham" *Cambria* **13** 151–180

GRO, 1988, "Estimated population at 30 June 1988: Scotland", General Register Office, Population Statistics Branch, New Register House, Edinburgh EH1 3YT

Hartnoll R, Lewis R, Daviaud E, Mitcheson M, 1985a *Drug Problems: Assessing Local Needs* Drug Indicators Project, Birkbeck College, Malet Street, London WC1E 7HX

Hartnoll R L, Lewis R, Mitcheson M, Bryer S, 1985b, "Estimating the prevalence of opiuid dependence" *The Lancet* 26 January, pages 203–205

Haw S, 1985 *Drug Problems in Greater Glasgow* Standing Conference on Drug Abuse, 1/4 Hatton Place, Hatton Garden, London EC1N 8ND

Herbert D T, 1982 *The Geography of Urban Crime* (Longman, Harlow, Essex)

Herbert D T, Smith D M (Eds), 1989 *Social Problems and the City: Geographical Perspectives* (Oxford University Press, Oxford)

Home Office, 1984 *Prevention: Report of the Advisory Council on the Misuse of Drugs* (HMSO, London)

Home Office, 1989 *Statistics for the Misuse of Drugs in the United Kingdom, 1973–1988* Home Office, Statistical Department, Lunar House, Wellesley Road, Croydon CR0 9YD

Jones K, Moon G, 1987 *Health, Disease and Society: An Introduction to Medical Geography* (Routledge and Kegan Paul, Andover, Hants)

Levy B, 1985 *Prevalence of Abuse of Substances in the Brighton Health Authority Area* Brighton Drug Dependency Clinic, Brighton BN1 3RA

MacGregor S (Ed.), 1989 *Drugs and British Society* (Routledge, Chapman and Hall, Andover, Hants)

Mann J M, Chin J, Piot P, Quinn T, 1988, "The international epidemiology of AIDS" *Scientific American* **259**(4) 60–69

Mather P M, 1976 *Computational Methods of Multivariate Analysis in Physical Geography* (John Wiley, Chichester, Sussex)

Mott J, 1981, "Criminal involvement and penal response to drug problems in Britain", in *Drug Problems in Britain: A Review of Ten Years* Eds G Edwards, C Busch (Academic Press, London) pp 217–243

Mott J, 1986, "Estimating the prevalence of drug misuse" *Research Bulletin* number 21, pages 57–60, Home Office, Research and Planning Unit, Lunar House, Wellesley Road, Croydon CR0 9YD

Mulé S J (Ed.), 1981 *Behaviour in Excess: An Examination of the Volitional Disorders* (The Free Press, New York)

NCC, 1983 *Disadvantage in Nottinghamshire: County Deprived Area Study, Part I* Nottinghamshire County Council, Trent Bridge House, West Bridgford, Nottingham NG2 6BJ

NCC, 1984 *Disadvantage in Nottinghamshire: County Deprived Area Study, Part II* Nottinghamshire County Council, Trent Bridge House, West Bridgford, Nottingham NG2 6BJ

Norliffe G B, 1977 *Inferential Statistics for Geographers* (Hutchinson Education, London)

O'Bryan L, 1985 *Adolescent Research Project: Interim Report to the DHSS* Drug Indicators Project, Birkbeck College, Malet Street, London WC1E 7HX

OPCS, 1982, "Small area tabulations", Office of Population Censuses and Surveys (HMSO, London)

OPCS, 1988, "Resident populations at mid-year, 1987: England and Wales" Office of Population Censuses and Surveys, Segensworth Road, Titchfield, Fareham PO15 5RR

Parker H, Bakx K, Newcombe R, 1986 *Drug Misuse in Wirral: A Study of Eighteen Hundred Problem Drug Users Known to Official Agencies* Sub-Department of Social Work Studies, University of Liverpool, PO Box 147, Liverpool L69 3BX

Parker H, Newcombe R, Bakx K, 1987, "The new heroin users: prevalence and characteristics in Wirral, Merseyside" *British Journal of Addition* **82** 147–157

Pattison C J, Barnes E A, Thorley A, 1982 *South Tyneside Drug Prevalence and Indicators Study* Centre for Alcohol and Drug Studies, St Nicholas Hospital, Newcastle upon Tyne NE3 3XT

Pearson G, Gilman M, McIver S, 1987 *Young People and Heroin: An Examination of Heroin Use in the North of England* (Gower, Aldershot, Hants)

Peveler R C, Green R, Mandelbrote B M, 1988, "Prevalence of heroin misuse in Oxford City" *British Journal of Addiction* **83** 513–518

Plant M, 1989, "The epidemiology of illicit drug use and misuse in Britain", in *Drugs and British Society* Ed. S MacGregor (Routledge, Chapman and Hall, Andover, Hants)

Redfield R R, Burke D S, 1988, "HIV infection: the clinical picture" *Scientific American* **259**(4) 70–79

Reed J L, 1980, "Drug dependence in contemporary societies", in *Environmental Medicine* Eds G M Howe, J A Loraine (William Heinemann, London) pp 270–280

Simpson A, 1981 *Stacking the Decks: A Study of Race, Inequality and Council Housing in Nottingham* Nottingham Community Relations Council, Mansfield Road, Nottingham NG1 3BB

Smith C J, Giggs J A (Eds), 1988 *Location and Stigma: Contemporary Perspectives on Mental Health and Mental Health Care* (Unwin Hyman, Winchester, MA)

Smith C J, Hanham R G, 1982 *Alcohol Abuse: Geographical Perspectives* (Association of American Geographers, Washington, DC)

Spear H B, 1969, "The growth of heroin addiction in the United Kingdom" *British Journal of Addiction* **64** 245–255

Thomas C J, 1971, "The growth of Nottingham's residential area since 1919" *East Midland Geographer* **5** 119–132

West L J, Cohen S, 1985, "Provisions for dependency disorders", in *Oxford Textbook of Public Health, Volume 2: Processes for Public Health Promotion* Eds W W Holland, R Detels, G Knox (Oxford University Press, Oxford) pp 106–137

Winchester H P M, White P E, 1988, "The location of marginalised groups in the inner city" *Environment and Planning D: Society and Space* **6** 37–54

Previous volumes in the series